# The Blackbird's Song

## and Other Wonders of Nature

A year-round guide to connecting with the natural world

# The Blackbird's Song

## and Other Wonders of Nature

A year-round guide to connecting with the natural world

## MILES RICHARDSON

NR

Published in 2025 by New River Books
www.newriverbooks.co.uk

10 9 8 7 6 5 4 3 2 1

A CIP catalogue record for this book is available from the British
Library.

Cover design by Smith & Gilmour
Cover artwork © Vanessa Bowman
Interior illustrations © Evie Dunne

ISBN: 978-1-915780-65-2

Printed and Bound in the UK using 100% Renewable Electricity
at CPI Group (UK) Ltd, Croydon, CR0 4YY

This FSC© label means that materials used for the product have
been responsibly sourced.

Excerpts from Richardson, M. (2012) *Needwood: A Year in
Search of Ordinary Things* and Richardson, M. (2014)
*A Blackbird's Year: Mind in Nature* appear with the permission
of the copyright holder.

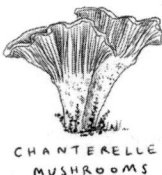

CHANTERELLE
MUSHROOMS

# Contents

**Preface**

**Introduction – A new way of being**
Natural wellbeing
What exactly is nature connection?
The pathways to nature connection
Learning to see
Nature and writing
*Activity*: Start a nature journal
A year ahead

**January**
Biophilia
*Activity*: What's your relationship with nature?
The joy of birds
*Activity*: Joy-watching birds
Trees are our closest neighbours
*Activity*: Get to know a tree
Angel: The blue tit
*For nature*: Provide homes and food for birds

**February**
Noticing nature
Three good things
What are the good things in nature?

*Activity*: Three good things for nature connection
Knowing nature
*Activity*: Read a classic nature writing book
Cold and the body
*Activity*: A frost walk
Angel: The blackbird
*For nature*: Provide or manage a wildlife pond

## March

Nature is our natural habitat
*Activity*: Go outside, be outside
The power of awe and wonder
*Activity*: Awe walk
*Activity*: Get to know a tree
Angel: The dunnock
*For nature*: Sow pollinator-friendly flowers

## April

The soft fascination of nature
*Activity*: Find and enjoy a blossom spot
What we eat
*Activity*: Grow your own
Lost words
*Activity*: Compile a nature playlist
Angel: The chiffchaff
*For Nature*: Do not disturb – people, pets and wildlife

## May

Forest bathing
*Activity*: Forest, woodland or park bathing

How nature manages our moods
Reflection
*Activity*: Reflecting on nature
Mindful attention
*Activity*: Mindful connection with birdsong
Angel: The swallow
*For nature*: Rest a mower and liberate your lawn

**June**
Flower power
*Activity*: Find a flower
Solstice and spirituality
*Activity*: Celebrate the summer solstice
Angel: The starling
*Activity*: Get to know a tree
*For nature*: Create homes for insects

**July**
The impact of technology
*Activity*: A trip into nature
The impact of becoming urban
*Activity*: Go on an urban nature safari
Blue spaces
*Activity*: Paddling on the shoreline
Angel: The swift
*For nature*: Take part in a butterfly count

**August**
Night and day
*Activity*: Go on a dusk walk
The long view
*Activity*: A social forage for blackberries

Creativity
*Activity*: Draw
Angel: Robin
*For nature*: Take part in a beach clean or litter
pick

## September

Landscape preference
*Activity*: Visit a viewpoint
Kinship with plants
*Activity*: Watch roots grow
Beyond being human
*Activity*: A kind of animism
Angel: The house sparrow
*For nature*: A log pile ecosystem

## October

Invisible friends
*Activity*: Breathe
Drama and song
*Activity*: A nature-inspired artwork
*Activity*: Get to know a tree
Angel: The rook
*For nature*: Be messy

## November

Virtual nature
*Activity*: Nature's gallery
Storytelling
*Activity*: Create a nature connection story
Maps
*Activity*: Make a nature connection map

Beyond the moment
*Activity*: Cherishing favourite moments from
    the past
*Activity*: Time walk
Angel: Long-tailed tit
*For nature*: Clean your nestboxes

## December
A friend in nature
*Activity*: Celebrate the winter solstice
The power of visualisation
*Activity*: Time travel
Keep on noticing
*Activity*: A Christmas craft walk
A nature-connected society
*Activity*: A vision of the future
*Activity*: Get to know a tree
Angel: The waxwing
*For nature*: Plant a native tree – and celebrate!

## Closing a year of connection

*Endnotes*
*Bibliography*
*Appendix and Further Reading*
*Acknowledgements*

# Preface

For 40 years I didn't realise I was disconnected from nature. As a child in the 1970s and 80s, I spent a lot of time outside – playing in the garden, over the road in the 'spinney', exploring fields, messing about down in the woods, or in the local brook. All sorts of activities – building dens, collecting frogs and snails, damming streams, floating boats, paddling and sometimes up to no good. I was very fortunate to have all these opportunities on the doorstep. I also went on family holidays, where I explored a wider variety of landscapes: the Lake District, Norfolk, Wales, Scotland, the Devon coast. I enjoyed being outside, sheltering from the rain and watching birds.

An ideal childhood to develop a close connection with nature? One would think so. Yet, I can see now that nature was an arena – a resource for recreation, something to divert and amuse me – while at the same time, I was being schooled and raised within a culture that had overseen the nation becoming one of the most nature-depleted in the world. Our free-roaming parents, grandparents and several generations before them were unwittingly part of the loss of our wildlife and habitats:

decades of gradual decline obscured by shifting baselines. We may think we're a nation of nature lovers – we believe in the beauty of our green and pleasant land, one celebrated by great poets and artists. But to really love nature, we need to connect with it, and this involves much more than merely roaming freely; it is a state of being, where we put nature first.

By the late 1980s, I was moving into the world of work; mundane weeks punctuated by weekends filled with the things we do to entertain ourselves and bring meaning to our lives – playing sport, joking with friends at the pub, taking photographs, listening to music, and yes, going for walks, enjoying nature. The possibilities seemed to increase year on year, each activity added into the mix of life to bring pleasure and satisfaction. Nature was just another enjoyable ingredient.

Two decades passed, during which I changed jobs, moved around, bought a first house, got married and had children. Again, any time I spent in nature I greatly enjoyed. And then, just over a decade ago, my relationship with the natural world underwent a profound change.

In January 2011, I started to wander the local pathways and modest green spaces on the edge of the suburbs where I live. I used my first smartphone to record my experience, simple sentences about the natural stimuli and my responses. In the course of 500 modest walks over two years, my notes grew from attentive observations into 100,000 words celebrating the joy of everyday nature and a personal reconnection to it. Through these trips and the simple act of writing itself, I stumbled on the universal story about our connection with nature. And ultimately this changed my understanding of my *self* and my shared place in the natural world. The experience led to me forming the first research group – at the University of Derby – with a direct focus on understanding and improving nature connection. The group has since undertaken dozens of projects, produced multiple research papers and formed several partnerships to implement our findings. It is this research and practice that underpin this book.

# A new way of being

A close connection with nature offers a way for both people and the natural world to flourish. Our wellbeing as humans is intricately tied to our relationship with nature, just as a fish needs water and a bird the air. We know this, deep down, and yet we seem to have set up our world to do the very opposite. Our consumerist society with its ever-increasing reliance on technology has effectively distanced us from the natural world. And the result is a decline not just in nature's wellbeing but in ours too. Many of us have noticed that there are fewer insects and fewer birds than there were when we were children. The signs of a changing climate are also becoming more apparent; we're getting used to hotter summers and wetter winters. An increasing lack of mental wellbeing completes this sorry tale. The three crises of biodiversity, climate and mental health are symptoms of our disconnect from nature, a failing relationship predicated on use and control rather than love and respect.

A new relationship with nature can start simply, but ultimately it is about a powerful new way of being. In this guide, I explain how to bring the wonder of nature into your everyday life in tangible and practical ways – with activities which, if maintained and embedded, will eventually change your perspective and your view of your place in the world. Along the way, I explain the benefits nature can bring, and outline the research and science that lie behind each activity.

The word 'everyday' is key here. My research over the past decade has confirmed the power of simple engagement with local nature – which is essential because we cannot all travel to wild places each day or live a rural life. A new way of being needs to be born close to home, in the fields, in the parks, in our gardens – wherever the blackbird sings.

From the simplicity of taking a breath to imagining a journey through time and being a good ancestor, this guide maps out a rich variety of ways to connect with nature. We will look at how the joy of birds or the gentle fascination of flowers restores us and helps manage our emotions; at the remarkable benefits of immersing ourselves in woodland or paddling along the shoreline. It is a guide that celebrates the natural year and the intricacies of a vital relationship that has become hidden by our busy lives.

## Natural wellbeing

Wellbeing is a common word, a catch-all for the various elements of our lives that contribute to our physical and mental health. At its heart, though, are two words: well and being. Wellbeing isn't just a pill to pop; it is a way of being well, all day, every day. A deep foundation for wellness.

A recent report on mental wellbeing across the world placed the UK second to last – only Uzbekistan did worse![1] Shockingly, a third of people in the UK reported being distressed or struggling, whether from low mood, an inability to regulate emotions, poor relationships or an imbalance between mind and body. The UK did perform better on resilience and drive, but as we'll see, even this points to our unbalanced state. Many of the 'core Anglosphere' nations, such as Ireland and Australia, were towards the bottom of the list, too.

By contrast, several Latin American and African nations topped the rankings, showing that greater economic development and wealth do not necessarily lead to greater mental wellbeing. For many decades in the UK, economic progress and prosperity have been delivered with the continual promise of greater happiness. The good times are always just around the next corner; each new technology a step towards fulfilment. How to explain, then, that, according to the survey, we would need an 86% improvement in mental wellbeing to reach the top spot?

Another piece of research throws a spotlight on the fact that our relationship with nature in the UK is particularly poor,[2] with most people not really engaging with or noticing it at all. Inevitably, this is affecting our wellbeing. People who are disconnected from nature – those who care less for the environment, or have a lack of wildlife nearby – have lower wellbeing. This is why the concept of 'one health', which encompasses both humans and the rest of nature, is important. We can't be healthy on a sick planet.

The good news is that we can do something about this. By making just a few changes in our lives, by realigning our daily habits to bring us closer to nature, we can reconnect – and this reconnection can bring not just joy and calm, but a much greater sense of wellbeing in general. When it comes to having a worthwhile and meaningful life, nature connection is four times more important than our socio-economic status.[3]

## What exactly is nature connection?

There are two key aspects to nature connection. First is the knowledge that humans are part of nature. We are not alien creations or elaborate robots or cyborgs; we are biological beings, mammals, apes. Second is a deep emotional bond with nature. And these two aspects interact. Nature connection is the realisation of our shared place in nature, and how we experience the world here and now – our feelings, beliefs and attitudes towards the rest of the natural world. Nature cannot be just a resource. As nature looks after us, we must look after it too.

So, nature connection is about much more than visiting and spending time in nature. People with a close connection with nature are likely to be in natural spaces more, but research shows that nature connection can increase without actually spending more time in it. It's about the *quality* of engagement during the time you're out in it. Nature connection is a mindset – a deep and meaningful relationship that involves both heart and mind and in which the lines between human and nature dissolve.

As we'll see in more detail through the months ahead, a rapidly growing body of research shows that people with a close connection with nature not only feel happier and that their lives are more worthwhile; they are also more willing to take action to help wildlife and the environment. So nature connection can help address the crises in biodiversity and climate as well as mental wellbeing. Across the world, major institutions are realising the need for a new relationship with nature, and evidence reviews are promoting the solutions offered by the science of nature connectedness.

## The pathways to nature connection

Our research has shown that a closer connection with nature is built by actively and repeatedly engaging with nature in a variety of ways. We call the five different types of engagement 'the pathways to nature connection'[4], and they are as follows:

- *Senses*: noticing and actively engaging with nature through the senses. Looking, listening, touching, smelling and sometimes tasting nature.

- *Beauty*: seeking out, appreciating, engaging with and celebrating the beauty of nature. Arts-based activities like painting, photography or writing are great ways to follow this pathway.
- *Emotions*: engaging emotionally with nature. Noticing the feelings nature evokes, from calm and wonder to joy and delight.
- *Meaning*: exploring and expressing how nature brings meaning to our lives. From our individual stories to nature's representation in the arts and cultural events, such as celebrating the summer equinox.
- *Compassion*: caring and looking after nature. Taking actions that protect and support nature, such as creating homes for wildlife, joining conservation organisations and rethinking our shopping habits.

## Learning to see

The pathways to nature connection provide a broad framework to return to, and all the activities in this book tap into them in one way or another. The broad aim is to help us form an emotionally meaningful relationship with nature. Our schooling and mindset have led many of us to believe that knowing the facts and figures about the natural world are the key to a caring relationship. However, reducing nature to parts and labels can keep us one step removed from real engagement. In addition to presenting the science, this guide includes activities that engage the emotions. But first, let's consider some more general ways of being.

## Doing less and seeing more

With busy lives, time can often dictate the day. Even when setting out to connect with nature, we're conscious that we'll be compelled to leave. Having to keep checking the time is unhelpful, so take your trips when you know they will fit comfortably into the time available. This approach will help you to be 'in the moment' and enable a mindful wandering away from intrusive thoughts so you can experience the world around you in an open and accepting way. Over time this can develop into mindful awareness, a deep knowing and freedom of mind that enhances the sensory impact of nature.

## The local landscape

The local area is the most practical and sustainable location for connecting with nature. Indeed, the benefit of staying local is that it can be done in small pockets of time. You can do less and start to see a little more. If you feel that you can walk out into nature straight from your door, be this along tree-lined asphalt foot-paths, or through leafy neighbourhoods or parks, you will be more likely to make regular trips. Which is doubly rewarding: nature that is frequently and closely observed soon becomes familiar, yielding new stories each day. Even in the most built-up areas wilderness can be found within a single bloom.

Try also to locate a few places in the vicinity that have a little more nature; look at a map, investigate the footpaths and find places you want to return to. When I find new places, I often feel compelled to return again and again. I once wandered a new path on six consecutive days until I felt I understood the place and had become familiar with what it had to say. Pathways allow more than just travel between locations; they provide ways to wander without the need for thought. Pathways reduce distractions, the need to make decisions, think and plan. The trouble-free ground liberates the gaze and allows effortless attention to the surrounding nature. Pathways allow mindful progress.

Either way, try and make life easy for yourself. Seek out ordinary nature, the wildlife that presents itself to you, the trees and flowers in your local park – even something growing in a gap in the pavement. Each spot has its own wilderness to discover. Animals are more difficult to glimpse – many are active at night and most shy away from human contact. Birds, however, sing their presence and are usually quite visible because they find security in the sky. Look out for the way the light catches their wings and the patterns of their song and flight.

Whatever your approach, do not become overly concerned with identification and analysis, and certainly not to the point where it distracts you from the fascination of form and movement. Yes, it is nice to know an ash from a rowan, or a redwing from a thrush, and it is worth becoming more aware of these facts. Knowing that the blackbird sings for only half the year, for example, is helpful when you are trying to be curious about nature, to see it with new eyes. But leave these discoveries for when you return home, or your precious time in nature can be lost to reference.

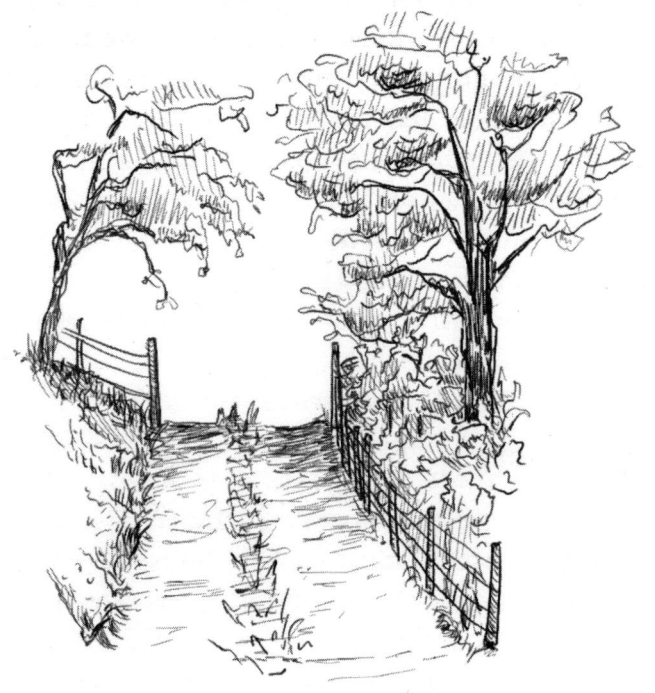

### The story of the day

Nature always has a story to tell and developing a connection with it is in many ways learning to read those stories. Each step is another word in the story of the day. Each passing bird and leaf unfurled is a new sentence.

Allow nature to speak to you; consider what you hear, see and feel. Time is another storyteller, allowing us to get to know nature, from dawn (which I achieved once!) to dusk (my regular companion).

And then there is the weather – a constantly changing backdrop. It's not always possible to ensure that our forays outside coincide with good weather. So you will experience everything the elements have to offer. Try and turn this into a positive. Engage with the different conditions, as they bring change to the familiar. The quality of light, the presence of mist or rain, the tug of the wind are all there to be understood more fully. Depending on what time you venture outside, and what the weather is doing, your local area will be constantly redescribed, creating a story of the day to grab and enjoy.

The landscape can also tell of stories past. Locations and plants can trigger recollections from previous walks, and different moods: the gate where the fox cubs played, the pond on that day with its exhilaration of swifts or the post where the barn owl perched. Each path, plantation and tree, each flower and bird, is connected to another time; each scent and reflection, each cloud and gust of wind, both a present connection and a memory of the past, which help you to weave your *self* into the landscape.

Just as getting an aerial view – having previously only seen things from the ground – can reveal the landscape in a new way, when we travel to unusual heights of engagement, we can see nature anew, and read new stories in it. Exciting stories, and stories that give us a sense of release, but also stories that make us aware of the kindness and wisdom of nature, how it seems to 'know' and have complete understanding of everything. We may experience a shift of awareness and emotion, as we undertake a new journey within a familiar landscape.

## Nature and writing

As we relearn how to look, how to see and 'read' each day with our senses, we can deploy another crucial tool to amplify the voice of nature: writing.

There is a long tradition of writing about the natural world. Hundreds of years ago, writers such as William Wordsworth and Richard Jefferies recognised how the emerging modern age was creating a growing divide between humans and nature. The continuing celebration of their work demonstrates that nature still means a great deal to people.

We perhaps all wish our lives to be meaningful, and writing can be seen as a search for meaning. This may seem very deep and challenging, but it's a simple reason to write, rather than required practice. Research evidence suggests that we don't need to write novels – regularly writing a few short positive lines for just two minutes a day can bring health benefits such as increased happiness. Longer expressive writing, which can be as little as five minutes a day, about our deepest thoughts and feelings, can help reduce negative emotions and benefit mental health. Across all ages, personality types, cultures and genders, writing that includes positive emotions makes the most difference. For humans, constructing stories is a natural activity that helps us process our experiences and better understand ourselves. Writing brings coherence and meaning, making the emotional effects of whatever we are going through more manageable.

The act of writing shouldn't be seen as a substitute for speech, or as an act of record or transferring knowledge, but an activity that shapes and enables thinking. Writing is thinking in action. Writing makes meaning. Add in the influence of nature on having a meaningful life and one can see the power in writing about nature. Writing about nature helps unite the mind and the natural world. This might seem like deep philosophical stuff, but it is very real. I could turn to scientific terms such as writing being 'embodied cognition' and refer to theories of 'extended mind' where our bodies and the 'external' world work together to such an extent that they aren't really separate. But let's leave it there for now because the simple act of noticing nature and jotting our observations down should be just that – simple.

### *Activity*: Start a nature journal

Writing is a great way to fully connect with nature, and the New Year is an excellent moment to begin, the dark evenings providing a time to reflect on your day's moments with nature. Or to revise the notes you've made 'on foot'. Firstly, some essentials:

- There are no rules!
- Buying a blank notebook is a wonderful way to start if you want to keep it natural, authentic and beautiful.
- Our ever-present smartphones can also become a tool for connection, enabling you to type as you go or dictate and make use of speech-to-text apps.
- Start close to home – either with the view from your window, or in your garden or local park.
- Give yourself a little time to look around and notice plants and wildlife, take time to sit or stand, a few days a week ideally, even if it's only for a few minutes.
- Don't worry about mistakes. This is your personal record.

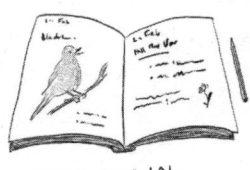

NATURE JOURNAL

There are many good guides to creative writing or to writing well, but that is not the aim here. This first activity is simply to start writing down what you see and think about during your moments in nature and ideally to keep doing that through the year. There is no need to get bogged down in identifying everything or to worry about the quality of your writing – although of course the process of reading and review can be enjoyable, giving you an end product that you might like to return to, or share.

We've covered how for me, short, local walks, writing as I went, were key to my reconnection with the rest of the natural world. The start of my writing was very basic observation. The notes below from day one are somewhat dry and descriptive as I forced myself simply to note down the things around me.

*A blanket of blue grey cloud*
*Low sun begin to feel warmth*
*Picking out colour in reeds and lumps of grass*
*Lightest breeze*
*Mud*
*Frozen*
*Pond still iced*
*Shroud of fog lifted*
*Tweet of unknown bird*
*Lone rabbit*
*Blackbirds*
*Such a peaceful crisp end to a short winter's day*

Jotting down simple cues like this while on foot are useful, as there are times when the writing should not break the moment. For me, these cues were enough to inform more reflective writing later in the day. The final order often matched the real timeline, but there are no rules. That first day became:

*After a day beneath a static blanket of blue grey cloud, brightness came and there was time to begin my search for ordinary things. At Anslow Park the sun, our ordinary star, was low in the sky and intensely reflected in the pond that had been frozen for a few weeks. It extracted and teased the remnants of colour from the reeds. Attentive, I sensed the faint breath of cold air flowing through the hedgerows. Occasional birdsong could be heard, a lone rabbit ran into the field and two blackbirds passed through the young trees in front of me.*

As I progressed through the year, my notes often remained brief, but increasingly started to include short phrases that would come to me close to their finished form. And often these phrases would provide a theme for the trip. Importantly, the writing does not need to be prose; it can be a single sentence, poem or haiku. Although don't imagine that these require less time! For me, trying to condense a lot into a sentence or short poem required almost more thought.

*Like a flake of summer, a butterfly skittered along between the trees as the thistledown floated calmly, looping with the breeze. From their distant perch, hidden rooks bled their calls into the air of the changing season.*

These short sentences carry our thinking process and can help us create new ideas about our relationship to nature. So, write as much as comes naturally. It is not the quantity and quality that matters, but the process and attention given. After all, writing is not your primary aim – the purpose is to develop your enjoyment and appreciation of nature. That said, many writers find that walking helps them gather their thoughts, so the combination of engaging with the joys of nature and committing them to the page will hopefully mean time disappears and words flow as you become deeply immersed. My personal experience of doing regular nature-noting walks never felt like toil.

Writing is powerful. It encourages self-reflection, enabling access to aspects of our being that can further deepen a connection with nature. And as we have already noted, writing helps process and release emotions. Add in the fact that nature helps lift our mood and you can understand how keeping a nature journal can be so therapeutic, reducing stress and promoting mental wellbeing. All in all, writing is a route not just to a new relationship with nature, but to a new relationship with ourselves, supporting personal growth and bringing a sense of accomplishment and self-esteem.

## A year ahead

Although this guide starts in January you can begin your search for nature connection at any time of the year. Some of the activities are tied to a month, event or season, but many can be undertaken at any time or throughout the year. Adapt the activities so that they work for you.

Each month, I share the science of nature connection that informs each activity and tell a story of the human–nature relationship, whether this means stepping back and considering our ancestors, the wider landscape and our culture, or looking towards the future and thinking about urban living, technology and the mysteries of time itself. Each month also features a 'For nature' activity – a prompt to give back to nature as well as take pleasure from it. A sustainable future depends upon uniting our wellbeing with the wellbeing of nature so that they are indivisible. These 'For nature' activities are selected from a list reviewed by 70 conservation experts for their ecological impact.[5] Caring for nature brings it closer, and provides comfort and hope.

As you wander the pathways to nature connection, give your relationship time to develop. Like any relationship, it requires some dedication. Eventually, you should see yourself as being part of a larger web of life with a sense of shared belonging and embeddedness in the natural world. Pause regularly during your busy life and the power of nature will bring its gifts.

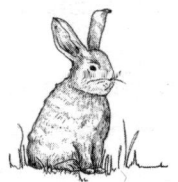

# JANUARY

Getting close to nature in January can feel like a challenge. Typically, it is the coldest, greyest and dampest month of the year in the UK, with short days and long nights. The trees have lost their leaves and it is a time of dormancy for many plants and animals. It is a great month to learn and develop new skills – how to look, to listen and to be.

With much of nature at rest, we need to be alive to the opportunities for wonder. The ever-present song thrush should be in song. And of course, there's often a robin about to brighten a winter's day. But winter also brings many visitors. Birds such as redwings and fieldfares will have migrated to the UK from the Continent to feast on berries. A few flowers emerge, such as snowdrops, winter aconites and perhaps lesser celandine. You may see lichens growing on rocks, trees and other surfaces. These hardy organisms, made up of algae and fungi, are an example of symbiotic relationships within the natural world. They appear lifeless, but can create miniature, alien-like landscapes to explore.

Nature's hidden presence can be revealed by tracks and signs. Look for feathers or fur on the ground, footprints in the mud or gnaw marks on trees. And when it's dark, as it often is in January, clear winter nights are ideal for lifting your gaze towards the stars.

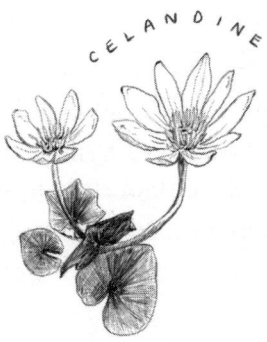

My own nature journal notes from a January over a decade ago show my search as I took my initial steps to a closer connection with nature:

*On this January day by the River Dove, the colour of the alder, spirit of the ash and static vigour of the hawthorn circuited the oxbow lake and all seemed content to rest as I watched the dance of the willow. The stillness of the water allowed me to look both down and up through its wonder of movement. Close by, the tree I'd named the painter's alder leant over the oxbow, forever reaching for its own reflection. Its trunk was as bright and curved as the neck of the swan that swam below; every angle explored*

*in its balance, as it paused on the bank like*
*winter's time.*

## Biophilia

You may well have heard of 'biophilia'; it's a concept that was popularised by Edward O. Wilson in a book of the same name published in 1984. Biophilia refers to our innate affinity for living things and the connections we subconsciously seek with nature for both survival and fulfilment.

The American ecologist Stephen Kellert further developed our understanding of biophilia by identifying nine values of the human–nature relationship.[6] It should be said here that, although often likened to a love of nature, biophilia is not all positivity. And Kellert's nine types of human–nature interaction also include aspects that have had or are having a negative impact and contributing to its decline – things like our utilitarian use of natural resources, our dominion and control –and even fear – of nature.

Of course, all animals use nature to survive and take action to avoid the dangers of the natural world, but sadly, many human populations have made excessive use of it. The nine values are a helpful way of drawing our attention to this skewed relationship. Growing fruit and veg purely for consumption, for example, especially when using pesticides to control 'pests', does little for nature connection; whereas organic gardening – ideally involving a bit of time to pause and enjoy the robins and worms – is likely to encourage a closer relationship.

### *Activity*: What's your relationship with nature?

Take a moment to consider each of the nine values of biophilia listed below. Consider how they are reflected in your own life and experiences with nature. You can also write down your thoughts and observations in your nature journal.

- Utilitarian. Nowadays, few of us are directly involved in meeting our daily needs through growing food and chopping firewood. Think about the practical uses of natural resources in your everyday life – everything from power and fuel, products and technology to food, for you and your pets. How much of this depends on natural resources? Much of our use of nature happens indirectly and depends on decisions taken by companies and corporations.
- Scientific. Consider your interest in studying and observing nature, whether it be from books or social media or television documentaries. Does this knowledge and understanding also cause awe and wonder in you, and contribute to the greater meaning of nature for you?
- Control. Consider your attitudes towards controlling and dominating nature. Do you have

a desire to tame and shape the natural world around you? Do you use chemicals to control 'weeds' and 'pests'? Are pesticides and weed-killers used to produce the food you eat?

- Fear. Explore your feelings towards and tolerance of nature. Are there things that evoke fear? Spiders? A dark wood on a misty day? Being stung by nettles or insects?
- Senses. To what extent each day do you engage with nature through your senses? What activities allow you to actively notice and engage with nature?
- Emotion. How does nature affect your moods each day? Which aspects of nature evoke positive emotions, such as joy and calm?
- Beauty. Contemplate how you find beauty in nature. What elements do you find aesthetically appealing?
- Meaning. Consider how nature brings meaning to your life each day. Perhaps it reminds you, in a positive way, how small we are within the web of life – this can help us get things into perspective. How often do you celebrate the natural world?
- Compassion. Consider what you do for nature each day. What steps have you taken to support and protect the natural world, both close to home and further afield?

By reflecting on the nine values, we can gain a deeper understanding of the various dimensions that form our relationship with nature. And this is important, because with much of our impact on the natural world hidden, the positive connections tend to be more visible, thus distorting our view. You may not ever really have thought of your relationship as utilitarian, for example – few of us set out to directly exploit nature – but you are likely to benefit from the industrial use and control of it. The sobering truth is that for the past five decades no country in the world has met the basic needs of its people without overconsuming natural resources.[7]

## The joy of birds

Birds are an ever-present face of nature in the modern world, both in reality and symbolically. Birds represent freedom, strength and peace. Their flight has long been associated with the human aspiration to break free from our earth-bound limitations and reach for the stars, while their migrations and new beginnings each spring are a symbol of hope and renewal. Some birds have their own unique meanings: the strength of the eagle, the wisdom of the owl. In many cultures, birds are seen as messengers from the spirit world or from ancestors, their presence and calls offering signs and omens. Birds appear regularly in religious texts; for example, the dove of peace and the impure raven in the Bible and the hoopoe, Solomon's loyal messenger, in the Quran.

Beyond symbolism, the presence of birds in our lives brings wellbeing. The richer and more various the birds in a neighbourhood, the higher people's satisfaction with life. Birds are one of the most loved class of creatures in nature. Birdsong is the natural sound linked most strongly to reducing stress and promoting restoration, particularly when it is more diverse and people are prompted to notice it. Birds bring joy.

### *Activity*: Joy-watching birds

A nature journal, while enjoyable and fulfilling, takes some effort and dedication. To watch birds all you have to do is sit back, let nature take the lead and focus on the happiness the experience may bring. There's no need for a pair of binoculars or a guide to bird species; we're not birdwatching in the traditional sense, although of course this is allowed! Clearly, birds need to be present, either through your window, in the local park or in the woodland or fields near where you live. See this month's 'For nature' activity for some tips on bringing birds closer to you. The only other requirement is to be comfortable and free from distractions; this is your simple moment with birds.

Joy-watching birds is about taking delight in their presence, their movement and their actions. Appreciating their community and vitality. Spend 30 minutes, allowing yourself to be enchanted by the wonder of flight and the joy nature offers for free.

To help maintain the focus on joy, rate your feelings for each species on a scale from one to ten. As I say, there's no need to get bogged down by identification at this stage; feel free to guess or make your own name up for now. Birds are more than their names and it is hard to develop a sense of nature connection if your experience is hampered by searching for the correct labels. There is plenty of time for learning which is a starling and which a sparrow.

Focusing on the joy of the activity is also better for your mental health. In our studies, when we compared joy-watching birds to identifying and counting them, we found that the people who simply focused on the joy of it had the greatest improvement in wellbeing.

To end the activity, take a moment to reflect on your joy ratings. Which birds topped the charts? Which birds did you struggle to appreciate? In our research, we found smaller birds tended to bring more joy, as did more colourful birds. We found corvids, like crows, rooks and jackdaws, got the lowest ratings, bringing around half as much joy as their smaller cousins. This returns us to where we started and the symbolism and meaning we attach to nature. Corvids have symbolic significance across many cultures. They are often associated with wisdom, intelligence and transformation. However, their black plumage has been linked to the underworld and even death in some cultures. Some see them as a pest, and these negative cultural associations have an impact on the emotions they evoke.

## Trees are our closest neighbours

Like birds, trees are usually present in our daily life. They too have a deep and varied symbolism, inspired by their longevity, deep-rooted strength and beauty. Growing from a tiny seed to a majestic giant before a slow, or sudden, decline, trees can represent the arc of life itself. They can also be seen as the silent observers of our lives, witnesses to human history, the repositories of time, wisdom and guidance. Their branches mirror those of a family and its ancestry – the tree of life.

Trees can carry a nation's values. They also feature in various religions and spiritual traditions; for example, the Tree of Life and the Tree of the Knowledge of Good and Evil in the Garden of Eden. In Buddhism, the Bodhi tree is a powerful symbol of enlightenment and spiritual awakening. Trees can be the dwelling places of spirits and symbols of interconnectedness. Like birds, trees have strong cultural associations. Cherry trees can represent beauty, olive trees peace and oak trees strength. The weeping willow can be linked to sorrow, or in some cultures flexibility and grace.

And again, as with birds, their presence is good for people, calming us and reducing stress. Even a view of at least three trees from a window can bring greater nature connection and wellbeing.[8] In addition to boosting our mental health, trees provide multiple environmental benefits, offering shade, improving air quality and reducing flooding.

In a recent study, the relationship between people

and trees was found to have three broad aspects: trees inspire admiration, they are seen as nurturing and they induce feelings of nostalgia.[9] In turn, these ideas reflect emotional connections, particularly when it comes to large and charismatic trees. People care about trees; they fight to save urban trees or local woodlands and mourn their loss. And trees play an important part in people's memories, their nostalgia for them implying a connection to something bigger than themselves.

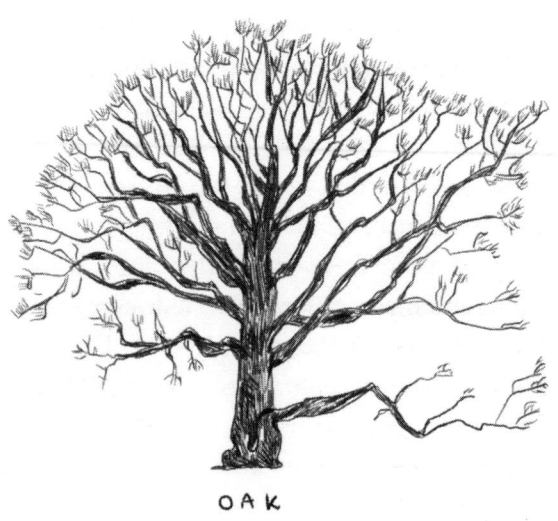

OAK

In our own research, we've been exploring how people value trees. In one survey, over 80% of people said they took notice of trees wherever they were, and 75% felt that large and noticeable trees were important to them. Around half of those we surveyed said they had a 'favourite tree'. Do you?

Interestingly, although many said they noticed trees and even had a favourite, few felt they had a very close relationship with them. (That said, the number of people who did feel close to a tree was double the figure for those who felt that they had a close relationship with their neighbours!)

### *Activity*: Get to know a tree

Make getting to know a tree a running theme across the year in your nature journal. This activity will serve as a tangible marker of the passage of the seasons and will help deepen your connection to nature.

Start by finding a local tree you'd like to get to know month by month, one that beckons, can be touched, or that will provide shelter or shade through the seasons. It may be a favourite tree already that you can explore further. Your chosen tree will hopefully become a regular companion for the year ahead. A deciduous tree would be best – it is much easier to track the seasons on a tree that loses its leaves than on, say, an evergreen fir. In January, you can begin by introducing yourself to the tree. Take a moment to trace it with your eyes from base to top. Let your gaze climb the trunk and explore how each branch divides, again and again, until the bare branches and twigs divide into air. Take in the tree's silhouette against the winter sky, its shape and form. Note down your favourite thing about the tree and see how it changes through the year.

## Angel: The blue tit

Birds survived the extinction of the dinosaurs and are a vestige of life from another age. Angels are messengers, and to me birds are angels from prehistory, their survival across millions of years reminding us of the resilience and adaptability of life and that we, too, can find ways to change and live more sustainably: birds have a voice and message we should listen to. For each month of the year I've selected an angel, usually a bird that is easy to find.

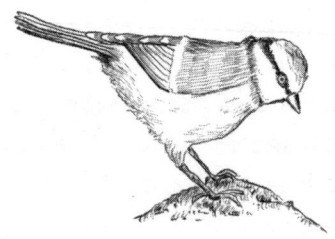

The blue tit is the angel for January, a lively, nimble bird with blue and yellow plumage topped by an azure crown. During the cold months, while their natural food sources are still limited, blue tits are quick to seek out the nearest garden feeder, so they're usually easy to spot flitting back and forth from a nearby bush or tree. They need to eat enough during the short day to see them through the long, chilly night. They're constantly on the lookout, alert to any risks or opportunities.

Ideally, find a spot busy with blue tits. Watch their flight, movements and interactions, and the way they compete for a spot on the feeder. Place your mind among them, feel the urgency, enjoy the display. On warmer days, as spring comes closer, you may see them looking for suitable nesting sites. Maybe you'll see them beginning to defend their territories and singing to proclaim their presence; a sweet call of short, rapid notes that brightens a gloomy winter day. These colourful little birds provide a flourish of life and optimism just when we need it.

## *For nature*: Provide homes and food for birds

Joy-watching birds is easier if you bring them a little closer to you. If you are fortunate enough to have some outside space, be it a yard, a garden or shared area, providing food and water for birds is a straightforward and rewarding activity. Even if you don't, there are options. Near to where I live, a man cycles to a quiet layby each day to refill the birdfeeders that have been there for as long as I can remember; it's a marvellous spot to visit.

Ideally, we should provide a rich source of natural food in our gardens and parks, by planting native shrubs and creating an insect-friendly environment. More on that below and in future months, but here are a few tips for feeding birds now.

*Varied feeders and foods foster a variety of birds and emotions*

If you can, try to set up two or three feeders with a variety of foods to attract different bird species. One feeder might be sunflower hearts, which are popular with finches, while another could contain peanuts, which tend to bring in blue tits, great tits, greenfinches and maybe others. Adding a seed mix, suet and mealworms to the menu caters for yet more species, such as robins and sparrows. In January, high-energy foods like suet are useful to help birds stay warm. And don't forget the drinks menu, which is easy: a shallow bowl of water is all they need.

There is one caveat to providing birdfeeders, which is that regularly feeding birds can lead to certain species becoming dominant. However, in my view, the disconnect from nature is so bad for both people and wildlife that the net benefit is positive, at least until birds become more widespread generally.

*Regular cleaning*

It is important to clean the feeders regularly to prevent the spread of disease. This can feel a bit of a chore, especially when feeders are busy, but as we know, care and compassion are key pathways to a closer bond with nature.

*Provide a home*

Having attracted some more birds, you can provide a home for them by installing a nestbox or two. You can either do this in your own space or volunteer to set some up in a local park, sports club or community garden.

Different birds have different preferences, so be guided by the birds you see regularly. Over the years I've tried a few types of boxes and have had most success with those designed for blue tits and great tits. So, that's probably a good place to start. You can buy one or, if you're confident with a saw, drill and hammer, make one yourself (there are simple instructions available online). If you are buying one, you don't need to spend a great amount, but please note that the twee tiny boxes that are widely available tend to be too small.

The position of the box is important. Facing north or east is usually recommended. The key thing is it shouldn't face south into the hottest sunlight. The box needs to be a couple of metres off the ground in a spot less likely to provide a cat with easy access. Having a tree or bush nearby is a good idea, but a box on a bare wall can work well too. Beyond the nestbox, try to foster an insect-friendly environment, by avoiding pesticides and letting a portion of your garden grow naturally – or select a community space that meets these needs already. If you've got the time and resources for it, you could go the full mile and replace a non-native shrub or two with a native species such as hawthorn. Your new neighbours rely on insects, not seeds and peanuts, to feed their chicks!

# February

February is the last month of winter and can be wet and windy with chilly temperatures, but any bright and crisp days that do come are inspiring. As the month progresses, you will find cheering signs of spring ahead. On your favourite tree, buds will begin to swell – a welcome sign of the imminent return of vibrant foliage. February is also the month when hazel catkins appear. A few centimetres of fascination hanging in clusters, these 'tails' are male flowers ready to release pollen that will fertilise the female flowers. Leaves start to unfurl on willow trees and blackthorn could well be in blossom. The first hawthorn leaves will emerge as frogs start to spawn.

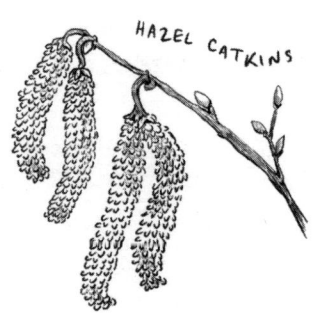

HAZEL CATKINS

Spring has been arriving earlier in recent decades – sometimes the first signs appear as early as February, a trend attributed to climate change. Of course, the arrival of spring varies across regions in the UK. For northern and inland regions, it arrives a little later. So, what's on offer will depend on your location.

As you wander in search of inspiration for your nature journal, you may hear rooks about their nests, and you'll see a few more flowers – early bloomers like crocuses and bright yellow winter aconites, forming a carpet on wide verges and woodland floors. On the coast, estuaries and mudflats teem with wintering waders feeding on the invertebrates exposed at low tide. And as the days gradually grow a little longer, birds become more audible, as they sing to establish territories and attract mates. Take a moment to be with them, consider their lives.

This short excerpt from my own nature journal shows the simple joys that can be found in February:

> *A bevy of long-tailed tits cracked and popped in the young oak above me, casting a dark shadow against the bark of the tree, kindly lit by the sun on this pure February day: everything edged by the brightness. A tall slender beech was shadowed with elegant curves by a neighbour, its branches sweeping upwards in compelling form to*

*make this one tree stand out from the many.*
*I felt replenished.*

## Noticing nature

Do you ever find yourself out in nature, but not truly engaging with what's around you? It's easy to pass birds and flowers without really seeing them or walk through woodland without paying attention to the trees. We can become so caught up in our own thoughts and conversations that we miss the sensory gifts that nature has to offer. Our research has found that some 80% of people rarely – or never – engage with nature by watching wildlife or pausing to smell a wildflower. Additionally, 62% of people rarely or never take a moment to listen to birdsong or notice butterflies and bees. Many of us have tuned out.

Tuning into nature via the senses can bring an important and long-lasting boost to our wellbeing. Think of it like this: when a musician is out of tune with the rest of the band, it creates disharmony and discord. So too when we are out of tune with nature, our lives are poorer for it. Furthermore, when we are tuned out, we fail to notice the state of the natural world. And, as we all know, noticing the problem is an essential step to taking action.

'Noticing nature' is about actively engaging our senses. This doesn't have to take time; moments with nature can come while doing other things. By tuning into the sights, sounds, and sensations around us, by listening to the birds, we can transform passive wandering into an immersive experience. When we truly notice nature, something magical happens. We start to appreciate its beauty, find meaning in its existence and feel a positive change in our emotions.

In the spring of 2020 when lockdowns restricted other activities, many more people started to wander about in their local patch and experienced a rise in their sense of wellbeing. In the UK, visits to nature increased by around 40%. Interestingly, though, our analysis of this data revealed that people's feelings of having a worthwhile life were not explained by the additional visits they made. Rather, it was to do with the increase in their noticing of nature which actually improved by over 70%.[10] The slower pace of life and lack of other distractions had led people to engage with nature more fully, boosting connection and the benefits that brings for wellbeing and pro-nature action.

This mirrors other research that shows the importance of noticing nature for building nature connection. What you do when out in nature – simple things like listening to birdsong and watching wildlife – is more important than the amount of time you spend there. Nature connection is about moments, not minutes. Clearly, moments require time, but the key is engagement. When stepping into a room of people, moments of connection come through talking to them, interacting, swapping stories.

Since 2020, our busy modern lives have returned,

with all their urban demands and digital distractions. The simplest way to break free from these demands and bring a sustained boost to nature connection is to notice the good things in it. It's a straightforward activity that can fit in with the busiest lives.

## Three good things

You may have heard of the idea of writing down three good things that have happened each day. Counting your blessings in this way has been found to improve wellbeing in many studies. Driven by my own experience of rediscovering a connection with nature by simply noting down what I saw, heard or encountered on my forays outdoors, I decided to make the 'three good things' nature-based. Indeed, 'noticing three good things in nature' each day was the first nature connection activity I developed, and the first to demonstrate sustained benefits.

The concept is super easy, and provides a useful prompt not only for us to get outside, but also to focus on nature as opposed to the other facets of our lives or surroundings. We ran a week-long trial involving two groups: in one, the participants were asked to write down three good things of their choice each day, while in the other, they were asked to write down three things they had enjoyed in nature. We found that people in the first group tended to pick examples from work or their interpersonal relationships – and their stress levels actually increased! Whereas those who had to write down three good things in nature showed sustained and significant increases in nature connectedness.

A few years, later we ran the study again, this time using a smartphone app to prompt people and enable them to record the good things in nature for one week. Again, we found lasting increases in nature connection which led to mental health benefits that were clinically significant for those with pre-existing mental health issues. Other people to benefit more were those who had started out with lower levels of nature connection and tended not to visit nature much.

We've repeated similar research a couple more times, with the same results, the improvements in mental well-being being on a par with the benefits seen from mindfulness and cognitive behavioural therapy. The 'three good things in nature' approach has also been used in a successful trial in which doctors gave patients a nature prescription.

## What are the good things in nature?

With all this research, we found ourselves with thousands of sentences documenting the good things in nature. And, when we analysed them, several themes consistently emerged. A key theme was the sensory experience of nature. People expressed appreciation for the sounds, sights and smells they encountered, such as the rhythmic crashing of waves, the scent of flowers and above all the joy of hearing birdsong. Another key theme was a gratitude for trees. People recognised the importance of trees, especially those in urban areas, as a salient feature of the local landscape, providing as they do shade and beauty amid the grey of asphalt and concrete.

The dynamism of the natural world was also a common theme. People found joy and fascination in observing the gradual transformation of nature over time, such as the emergence of buds in spring and the growth of new leaves. They also valued their encounters with everyday wildlife: the simple movements of birds or the playful antics of squirrels chasing each other in the park.

Although views, skies and the weather also cropped up – an added layer of wonder brought by a walk in the summer rain, a beautiful view, or clouds floating by on a breezy day – people seemed to find more meaning, inspiration and connection in the living aspects of nature: the first primroses, a robin hopping about in the garden. Whatever the topic, however, the beauty and wonder of nature was a constant, whether breathtaking landscapes or the intricacies of a spider's web.

### *Activity*: Three good things for nature connection

Taking the time to pause and to notice nature is an essential step to reclaiming our inherent connection to the natural world, which is an essential part of being human and fostering a profound sense of belonging. So, let's try. Every day for the next week, write down three good things in nature that you notice each day. These could be the beauty of small things noted in a given moment – the song of a robin or the movement of a tree in the breeze, for example – or wider aspects that arise from experiencing the diversity and wonder of the natural world around you.

A few tips for noticing nature:

- Slow down. It's all too easy to rush from one task to another without tuning into the surroundings. Pause, take a breath and consciously tune into wherever you find yourself. Whether you are standing at the bus stop or on a clifftop, take a moment to focus on something natural within view.
- Engage your senses. Listen to the birds, feel the texture of leaves, inhale the aroma of flowers and bathe in the sunshine or a gentle breeze.
- Walk. We've found that noting three good things in nature has an even greater impact when combined with walking. Each step offers new perspectives, until sometimes your surroundings may suggest a place to pause and stand still. Let the landscape or local park speak to you; even in a bustling city, you can find pockets of nature to explore.

You can make notes as you go, or return to reflect on your day in the evening. Whatever works for you. I often combined the two, making notes brief enough so as not to break the moment but providing sufficient information to jog my memory when revisiting the experience later in the day. At a minimum, you'll have three sentences each day, but you may choose to turn the notes into a couple of paragraphs. Maintain this, and you will create a library of good things in nature, something you can access and use to travel to in time. Here are a few examples of the good things in nature people have written:

> *the wonder of a spider web on the bin.*
> *the sound of the sea breaking on the shore.*
> *the fetching orange belly of the slug that I removed from my lettuces.*

## Knowing nature

What is it, to *know* nature? The meaning of 'to know' is often defined as: '*to be aware of through observation, inquiry or information*'. This suggests that learning labels, facts and figures is required. But when it comes to nature connection, too much focus on facts and figures is a mistake, suggesting as it does that there is a separation between the person acquiring knowledge and the thing they are learning about. This is an objectivist way of learning. Clearly, not a route to love.

However, there is another definition of to know, which is: '*to have developed a relationship with*'. When it comes to knowing nature, this makes much more sense. A long-lasting relationship is built on noticing beauty, emotions, meaningful experiences – and caring.

For me, reading other people's writings about nature was an essential part of my personal reconnection journey. But it took me a while to find the sort of nature writing that particularly spoke to me. There is plenty of writing about nature out there that includes facts and figures, and of course this can be fascinating. There's also plenty of nature writing that is essentially memoir, telling a story about the author, with nature being the cure for the difficult situations life presents. Let's think about this for a moment. Being more interested in ourselves is a growing trend. As the state of nature has continued to decline, with so much wildlife being lost, our focus has increasingly been turned on ourselves. Likewise, the use of words related to the natural world has declined, while the use of the word 'me' has quad-rupled since the 1990s. Even song lyrics have transi-tioned from mainly being about others to being about the singer. A human-centred approach to life has taken hold, with human experience being the supreme source of meaning. This is reflected in the way people describe their experiences in nature – in suburban European-American societies, nature increasingly tends to be referred to as a backdrop to their activities rather than as the main event; compare this to Indigenous commu-nities, who speak more frequently of foraging, forest walks and medicinal plants.

This human-centric view is inevitably reflected in a lot of writing, but some wonderful examples of texts about nature connection do exist. A commonly acknowledged classic is Nan Shepherd's *The Living Mountain*, which focuses on the experience of knowing nature. It was considered so unusual at the time of writing, during the Second World War, that it went unpublished for decades. And when it did come out, 30 years later, it was seen as strange and remarkable. It still is.

In her book, Shepherd demonstrated a new thinking and philosophy that saw a truth beyond the objectivist and fractured worldview that dominates the modern world. It's a study of how our bodies are instruments that can be tuned and refined to gain a deeper understanding of our connection with the natural world. Shepherd shows how, when simply lying on a mountainside, finding joy in the perception of the natural world, each sense can become a route into nature's offerings. She uncovers a deep connection with the Earth, such that any sense of self dissolves and merges with nature, creating a spirit that can walk out of the body and into the landscape.

On the closing page, Nan Shepherd writes: '*Knowing another is endless ... The thing to be known grows with the knowing.*'

I have also found an affinity with the writing of the Victorian naturalist Richard Jefferies, who found intense joy and meaning in everyday nature close to home. Like Shepherd, Jefferies' writing extended the body into the landscape, highlighting the interconnection between the human observer and the rest of nature.

> *The grass sways and fans the reposing mind; the leaves sway and stroke it, till it can feel beyond itself and with them, using each grass blade, each leaf, to abstract life from earth and ether. These then become new organs, fresh nerves and veins running afar out into the field, along the winding brook, up through the leaves, bringing a larger existence. The arms of the mind open wide to the broad sky.*
>
> from *The Sun and the Brook*

His repeated journeys noticing nature revealed the unity of the human mind and nature and how we are made happy by the unconscious visceral experience of nature.

> *We are of the great community of living beings, indissolubly connected with them from the lowest to the highest by a thousand ties.*
>
> from *Nature and Eternity*,
> published posthumously in May 1895

*Activity*: **Read a classic nature-writing book**

The long evenings at this time of year are ideal for reading a nature-writing classic. My suggestions are:

- *The Living Mountain* by Nan Shepherd
- *The Peregrine* by J. A. Baker
- *The Pageant of Summer* by Richard Jefferies, available free on the internet through Project Gutenberg.

Of course, there are all sorts of other writers who have explored wilderness around the globe or Indigenous wisdom, but our route to nature connection is closer to home. Feel free to choose whatever authors you want, and perhaps inspire your own nature journal.

## Cold and the body

Stepping into cold air and onto frost-covered ground can provide a truly invigorating experience that extends beyond our senses. The freezing conditions affect the landscape and our own physiology, uniting the physical and mental world and facilitating a deep connection with nature as we experience the intricate relationship between our bodies and the wider environment.

As we take the first steps into the chilly surroundings, crisp air fills our lungs, stimulating our respiratory system and triggering a series of physiological reactions as the body prepares to maintain its core temperature. The blood vessels in our extremities constrict to prevent heat loss around vital organs, and the skin tightens. Our sympathetic and parasympathetic nervous systems are at work.

The sympathetic nervous system, which deals with drive and threat, triggers the release of hormones that promote an increased heart rate and a heightened state of alertness. Simultaneously, the parasympathetic nervous system, responsible for promoting a state of rest and relaxation, stabilises the sympathetic response, helping to maintain balance and calm in our bodies. An initial state of heightened preparedness thus gradually settles into one of tranquillity. Just this little bit of awareness of how our bodies work can help us realise that we are biological beings that respond to the wider landscape.

Frosty conditions are not only visually engaging and beautiful; the sight of our breath billowing out into a mist, the sensation of the cold air on our skin, together with the crunch of frost beneath our feet, are all reminders of our place within an intricate natural system.

### *Activity*: A frost walk

Next time there's a cold day, don't snuggle inside, embrace the opportunity to take a frost walk. Anticipate stepping outside with positivity and wonder and engaging in an invigorating experience. Cultivate your awareness of the intimate relationship between your body and the wider world and allow this activity to deepen your connection with nature.

Your frost walk can be any length you wish, from a wander around the yard to a circuit of the park, or a special trip a little further afield. Choose a location and conditions you're comfortable with. Remember to take care if it's slippery underfoot, and make sure you dress appropriately.

And then: enjoy! Take a moment to feel the cold air on your face and notice your visible breath. On frost-covered ground, savour the crunch of crisp grass or fallen leaves. Take notice of the delicate frost on leaves, the crystal-lined twigs, and the patterned puddles. Note how the frost accentuates the details and beauty of nature. Pause and listen to the stillness. And do jot down – or commit to memory –the good things in nature and consider your next entry in your nature journal.

## Angel: The blackbird

It's time to introduce February's angel, the blackbird. With their vibrant orange beaks and eye rings, and their black feathers sparkling in the sunlight, these birds stand in stark contrast to the muted tones of winter.

While many blackbirds are residents in Britain, some may arrive from elsewhere in search of more favourable conditions. And February, when natural food sources are still scarce, can be a challenging month for them.

A supply of suitable food such as suet and seeds in a garden, on the ground or a table, may attract black-birds. You'll also likely find them foraging for fallen fruits, berries and any invertebrates or insects they can find in parks and other open spaces around residential areas. Listen as the light fades and they dart for cover, their alarm call ringing out through the gloom.

With spring and their breeding season not so far away, male black-birds will be defending their terri-tories in preparation. They typically return to song to establish their presence early in the year. At first, you might hear just some soft calls and whistles. But stick with your search because their melo-dious tunes, sung out from a prominent perch at dusk, are very special, each note a stitch, every flourish a tie, to a closer connection with nature.

*For nature*: **Provide or manage a wildlife pond**

The end of February is a good time to plan and begin a wildlife pond. Depending on the weather, planting may need to wait a month or so; but you should be able to start digging, which is an excellent way to keep warm!

A wildlife pond, whether it be a modest bowl in your backyard or a pond in a garden, is a great way to give back to nature, and creates a fascinating new world on your doorstep. If you don't have access to a yard or garden, or don't want to introduce the risk of a pond for young children, you can look for opportunities for local nature conservation volunteering, which may involve creating new ponds or managing existing ones. This can be a wonderful way to connect with like-minded people and help build a nature-connected community.

The first step in making your own pond is to identify a suitable location. Ideally, it should be away from over-hanging trees and receive a few hours of sunlight each day – and be close to somewhere you can sit. There's a great deal of pleasure in whiling away an hour beside a pond, especially one you've created.

You can use a container, such as a bowl or a small tub. It just needs to be sturdy, watertight and large enough to allow some space for aquatic plants to grow. Also, keep in mind that a smaller container pond may heat up more quickly in direct sunlight. You may need to monitor it closely to maintain water quality, but it's possible to create a rewarding habitat for wildlife in a compact space.

If you're digging a hole for a pond, the size and shape is up to you, but try to provide a range of depths to cater to different species. Also, you'll need to line the hole with a pond liner. Search online for tips on selecting the correct size – it needs to be big enough to overlap the edges of the hole.

Next, fill your pond with water and allow it to rest

for a few days before adding plants. Aim for a variety of native aquatic plants that will make good homes for a variety of creatures. This should include a mix of submerged, floating and marginal plants to create diverse habitats. Be careful to avoid plants that are fast growing and can take over your pond. Again, you can find lots of useful information about all this online. Then sit back and watch as your pond becomes a thriving home.

# MARCH

March is a month of renewed energy and growth in the natural world and it begins to feel much more like spring, on sunny days at least. The rising temperatures and longer days offer many opportunities to witness the awakening of the natural world. Leaves appear on sycamore trees, with the hornbeam close behind. There are many more spring flowers and more trees are in blossom, bringing welcome colour to gardens and parks. If they haven't already come out, blackthorn hedgerows will flower and hawthorn leaves will appear, providing essential cover and nesting sites – just in time for the arrival of the few familiar birds of summer that return from their wintering grounds in March.

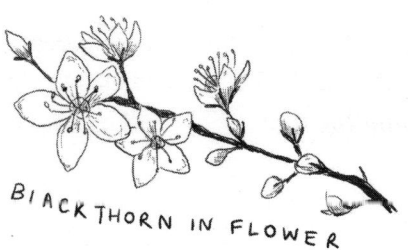

BLACKTHORN IN FLOWER

You should start to hear chiffchaffs call, and towards the end of the month sand martins appear. An ever-growing dawn chorus can be heard. Look closely enough and you may see basking reptiles and insects, alongside the first bumblebees, hoverflies, butterflies and ladybirds. It's an exciting time.

These nature journal notes of mine remind me of the feel of March:

> *March rose from the mists to engulf the landscape. Strands of gossamer web trailed from the hedgerow, revealed by the light like a slow-motion rain. The stark trees were compelling in their winter form, black against the bright sky, but I could sense the welling eruption of spring. Below the daytime moon, a pair of great spotted woodpeckers chased past. Trees sat like creeping vapours and only the nearby magpie was bold. The swans left the meadow to join the oxbow and gain more elegant motion. As smooth as the misted air, they rode the reflections of the now present sun as a skylark lifted to speak of spring, its speck floating against the blue, its accelerated song seeming to slow surrounding time.*

## Nature is our natural habitat

The fact that human beings have spent millions of pounds on research to establish the benefits of nature is one of the starkest signs of our disconnection from it. We readily accept, after all, that animals – from elephants to polar bears, meercats to penguins – are most suited to the natural world. Nature is their natural habitat; destroy that habitat, or remove a creature from it, and their wellbeing suffers. Why would this not be the same for us?

It's rarely mentioned, but humans are one of the great apes. We share brain structures and a biological continuity with them, and this includes similarities in vulnerability to stress and mental health issues. If chimpanzees, our closest living relatives, are removed from their natural habitat and placed in artificial environments, abnormal behaviours and disorders similar to those seen in humans can arise. Captive chimpanzees exhibit mental health issues like anxiety and obsessive-compulsive disorders, which are not typically seen in their wild counterparts. When chimpanzees kept in this way are returned to more natural environments, their abnormal behaviours decrease.

As creatures who evolved in the natural world and spent hundreds of thousands of years deeply embedded in it, we should readily accept that nature is inherently good, indeed integral to our health and wellbeing.

So, let's consider some of the benefits. Numerous studies have focused on the health differences between people living in rural and urban areas, and found that those in rural environments generally report better health compared to their urban counterparts. This passive exposure to nature has been shown to be important across many studies, with the presence and quality of local green spaces linked to lower rates of hypertension, nature providing a buffer against the negative effects of stress. Conversely, areas with fewer trees have been linked to respiratory and cardiovascular illnesses. The overall benefits are demonstrated by the fact that that people who live in greener neighbourhoods have longer 'telomeres', the structures that protect the ends of chromosomes, and which are linked to slower ageing of cells and longer lives.[11]

Even a simple view of green space can have benefits, with people reporting better physical and mental health and requiring fewer painkillers. Occupants of buildings with ample natural light and outdoor views have been found to have improved mood and better sleep quality.

Continuing this segue from physical to mental wellbeing, there is plenty of research establishing a positive link between nature and subjective wellbeing, i.e. the way we say we feel. Wellbeing includes things like positive mood, life satisfaction and vitality, which can in their turn lead to enhanced immune function. A positive relationship with nature also strengthens many of the functions of the brain, from perception and memory to reasoning and imagination, problem-solving and creativity.

Amazingly, passive exposure to nature has even been

found to have an impact on the structure of our brains. Deep within the brain, the amygdala plays a crucial role in processing emotions, and when over-active it can cause anxiety. There's evidence that simply living in areas with more trees benefits the integrity of this part of the brain.[12] Even though we may not consciously perceive the presence of nature, our deep, often hidden connection with it still has a profound impact on us.

Perhaps it's no surprise, then, to discover that higher levels of biodiversity, too, are linked to increased benefits, including greater positive emotional responses. People report being happier in places with a greater variety of birds and habitats – even if this is not the case, and they just *think* they are surrounded by an abundant diversity of nature. Our perceptions can matter more than reality.

From passive exposure, through simple engagement to close connection, the benefits of nature continue to mount. As we've seen, research has shown that a person's sense of nature connection can be four times more important than purchasing power in explaining their sense that life is worthwhile. Nature connection benefits have also been found to be similar in size to other established factors, such as marriage and education. Nature provides a restorative boost for body and mind. A strong sense of connection to it brings us happiness and satisfaction with life – a sense that life is worthwhile, and that we are flourishing!

## *Activity*: Go outside, be outside

This activity is very straightforward, but can be difficult to achieve in our modern lives, in which we spend around 95% of our time indoors, with just a few minutes close to green spaces each day. So, as spring arrives, and the weather warms a little, make a conscious effort to go outside and be outside. Here are a few hints, tips and simple ideas to help you incorporate this activity into your routine:

- Take your morning cup of coffee outside. Rather than rushing through your morning routine indoors, take a few extra minutes to enjoy your coffee in the open.
- Take a greener route to work, even if it's a little slower; explore detours that might take in a park or a leafy lane.
- Find a moment to go on a walk during your working day. If you have a one-to-one meeting or a brainstorming session with a colleague, suggest going outside for it. Remember, this can boost creativity and productivity too.
- Explore green spaces near your workplace. Discover nearby parks or outdoor seating areas where you can take a short break during the day or on your commute.
- Plan more outdoor activities. Use your free time to get outside, whether it's gardening, walking, cycling, sitting or litter picking.

- If you go to a café, take a coat and sit outside – but you might be surprised to find it's fine for the 10 or 15 minutes it takes to have a drink or snack.

The simple goal for this month and throughout the spring, summer and autumn is to actively seek out those extra moments outside each day.

## The power of awe and wonder

As we've seen, passive exposure to nature is good for us, but we can easily reap even more benefits from it through our expectations and outlook. Tapping into a sense of wonder when we're out in nature brings greater benefits than just walking or looking. Experiencing awe and wonder doesn't just make us feel good; it broadens our thinking and awareness, opening our minds to new ideas and allowing us to explore new possibilities and build personal resources that help us cope better with negative emotions in the longer term. It can reduce symptoms of anxiety and depression and increase prosocial behaviour, generosity and creativity, leading to a greater sense of connectedness with others and a greater sense of purpose in life. As ever, the boundary between mental and physical benefits blurs, with positive emotions bringing physiological benefits, such as reducing inflammation, improving cardiovascular health and boosting the immune system.

## *Activity*: Awe walk

Spring is the perfect time to go on a weekly awe walk. You don't need to make a special trip – awe can be found almost anywhere. Try to find something new in the familiar and make a conscious effort to adopt a childlike sense of wonder. There's natural wonder in a new leaf unfurling, for example. Or a bird flying. The scale of a large tree is incredible seen with fresh eyes.

Shift your attention beyond yourself, be in the moment and focus your attention on the wonder of nature. This may sound difficult, but with the right outlook it is easily done. In research studies, those who were found to benefit received no special training, just simple instructions like those above. The key is to trigger a sense of awe and immerse yourself.

## *Activity*: Get to know a tree

Back in January, you found a local tree to get to know month by month, providing a running theme through the seasons for your nature journal. How is that going? You traced the tree from base to top, letting your gaze explore its form against the winter sky. Remember to track the awakening of your tree as spring unfolds. Visit it regularly to witness the buds emerging and, depending on the type of tree, leaves unfurling. Track the changes each week and search for any other visitors as wildlife also explores your tree.

## Angel: The dunnock

March's angel is the dunnock. Little brown dunnocks seem to get little attention or celebration, yet they are reliable singers, in full voice through March like blackbirds, robins and thrushes. Dunnocks are common birds, with with streaky brown plumage and a grey head – subtle, but distinctive. You'll find them singing from a regular spot in parks, gardens, hedgerows and woodland. They are trickier to see when they're on the ground, probing leaf litter for insects, worms and spiders, or busily weaving together nests from twigs and leaves in some sheltered undergrowth. For me, this often-overlooked bird is a true angel, its spirited presence after winter a symbol of hope, renewal and determination.

## *For nature*: Sow pollinator-friendly flowers

A big problem for pollinating insects like bees and butterflies is a lack of flowers packed with pollen and nectar. So it's great to do what you can to provide some; and, if all goes well, you'll be rewarded with beautiful flowers and lots of insects to spot in the summer. Lazy summer days watching bees visiting your blooms are something to savour, especially when you do so knowing you're giving something back to nature.

*Choosing your seeds*

Late March is a little early for some seeds, but being ready means you won't miss the opportunity, and there's always some preparation required. You'll need a sunny spot that otherwise offers little for wildlife in your garden, or some containers. If that's not an option, perhaps a friend, relative or neighbour would be willing to benefit from your hard work!

Spend some time choosing some flower seed. You can consider native flowers suited to your local conditions, or non-native flowers that can also be beneficial for pollinators and bring added diversity. Here are some options for sunny spots with well-drained soil that should be relatively forgiving for beginners:

- Chives: very easy to grow, even in a patch of gravel. The flowers look great in May and the leaves can be used in cooking too.
- Aquilegia: attractive spring flowering plant that self-seeds to pop up in new positions each year.
- Phacelia: often called bee's friend, this purple, bell-shaped flower with abundant nectar is fantastic for attracting bees and other beneficial insects.
- California poppy: bowl-shaped orange and yellow flowers.
- Meadow cranesbill: a native purple flower of summer meadows.
- Nigella: also known as love-in-a-mist, this has delicate blue or white flowers in July and August

with feathery foliage. Can also manage partial shade.

- Thyme: a low-growing plant with tiny flowers that can even find a home in gaps between paving slabs.
- Lavender: fragrant purple blooms that attract bees and butterflies in July and August. 'Gros bleu' works particularly well.
- Catmint: very easy to grow and very popular with bumblebees from late spring to late summer.
- Marigold: cheery and strongly scented yellow and orange flowers.
- Marjoram: a native perennial with small purple flowers in July and August.
- Comfrey: excellent for bees, this very hardy plant flowers all summer.
- Knapweed: pink to purple blooms from June to September, a meadow wildflower that's well suited to the garden too.
- Sneezewort: small white flowers in July and August.

Finally, a few options that can tolerate a range of soil conditions:

- Lungwort: an easy early-spring option with bell-shaped flowers that does well in both sun and shade.
- Cornflower: attractive blue or pink flowers from May to September. Can also tolerate some light shade.

- Borage: bright-blue star-shaped flowers with a long flowering period and high nectar production.
- Field scabious: a native pale-blue meadow flower that blooms from July to September.
- Jacob's ladder: easy to grow, with clumps of small blue flowers around June.

Enjoy an evening reading up on the options, looking at photographs and listing your personal favourites. Remember that preferred growing conditions can vary a little depending on the region and climate. So, a little research or a conversation with an experienced gardener might be worthwhile to avoid disappointment and help you create a pollinator patch that's in bloom from spring to early autumn.

*Sowing your seeds*
As the soil begins to warm up from late March into April, you can follow a few simple steps to sow your chosen seeds:

1. Prepare the soil. In a location preferred by your chosen flowers, clear an area and lightly loosen the soil, sifting out larger stones, so that the seed can be sown and roots easily grow. If you are sowing seed in containers, make sure there are drainage holes before filling with potting compost.
2. Sow the seeds. Follow the instructions on the seed packets for the appropriate spacing and

depth. Lightly cover the seeds with soil and gently water them.

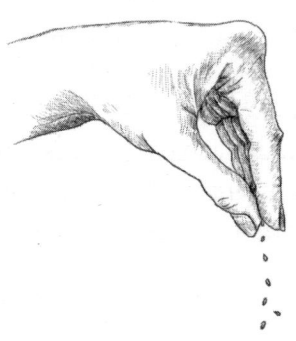

*Caring for your seedlings*
Your seedlings will need some TLC, so here are a few tips:

- Water. Keep the soil moist but not waterlogged with regular watering, especially during dry spells.
- Temperature. Be mindful of frosts or hot days. Cover your young seedlings or bring inside if necessary.
- Manage competition. Nature always finds a way and other plants will start to appear and compete with your seedlings. Pull them out and consider covering the bare soil with wood chippings or gravel to restrict regrowth. A living mulch such as clover or creeping thyme is another option.
- Monitoring. Check your plants for bugs or they

may become a food source for wildlife in an unintended way! Either let nature win and try another type of flower or consider organic options to protect your plants. Either way, it's a reminder of the ecosystem we exist within.

With proper care and a little good fortune, your chosen spot will become a small haven for bees, butterflies and other insects in the months ahead and provide lots of inspiration for your nature journal.

# APRIL

Spring accelerates through April as the longer and warmer days continue to bring further energy and growth. This creates many opportunities to take a moment to connect with the wonder of nature's awakening. The change is perhaps most apparent through the abundance of spring flowers and blossom. Gardens and parks are transformed by well-celebrated joys such as tulips, but don't neglect the humbler wildflowers, such as dandelions. Towards the end of the month, bluebells flower in some special woodlands, creating a real spectacle, while above them sycamore, beech and horse chestnut provide layers of greens. The buds on oak trees open to reveal the most vibrant hue. You'll find it much easier now to spot bumblebees, butterflies, such as peacocks and orange-tips, and the myriad of other insects that bring a buzz to spring and offer a feast for the senses.

With the warmer weather, it's much easier to be outside and find awe. Blue tits and blackbirds spend their days feeding their young before joining the chorus at dusk. Departed redwings and fieldfares are replaced by other bird species returning from their winter migration, such as house martins, swallows and willow warblers. Sadly, one symbol of spring in the UK is increasingly difficult to enjoy: the sound of the cuckoo, its call like a pulse of the landscape or a reminder of those lost. These birds are in worrying decline. Nature is resilient, but fragile and precious too.

These nature journal notes from April were born from walking and noticing:

> *April progressed and the skylarks were as constant as the air itself at Brankley, where the ground was sodden from weeks of regular showers. I circuited towards the young birch wood on the ridge above me, the trees coming into leaf once more and standing for attention. Their line became depth as I neared, until each unfurling leaf could be seen attached to bronzed and twiggy growth. Closer still, each leaf became a pair, cupped like hands, alternating to an end point and moving with the breeze.*

## The soft fascination of nature

You may have heard of a concept called 'Attention Restoration Theory', which explains how nature can restore us when we are suffering from the cognitive overload that comes with the constant stimulation of modern living. Nature's sights, sounds and textures can capture our attention in a unique and non-demanding way, providing a soft fascination that can foster an effortless sense of calm and help to restore our cognitive resources. Just 40 seconds of gently viewing nature can boost a fatigued mind. It frees us from the demands of having to pay attention and stay focused, allowing our brains to rest and recover, so we can return to improved performance and a state of wellbeing.

Our senses evolved to be able to comprehend the natural world, so it stands to reason that nature soothes, rather than strains and provokes, as it flows through us. We are primed to be able to tune into nature, our brains effortlessly processing its patterns, rhythms and beauty. This is not to say that nature is simple. On the face of it, nature's coherence and harmony may seem straight-forward, but there's a complexity and depth to it often not found in the manufactured products of our human world. Get closer and zoom into the enormous diversity in any natural scene; nature keeps giving, with ever-evolving layers of variation and form.

### *Activity*: Find and enjoy a blossom spot

It's April and what provides better soft fascination than blossom? From fruit trees to hawthorn hedges, spring is replete with it. In Japan, people enjoy the soft fascination of blossom every spring in a festival called *Hanami* (literally 'flowerviewing'). It has deep cultural significance as a symbol of the beauty and transience of life.

The blossom forecast is announced each day, encouraging people to gather and celebrate the trees in bloom, the fleeting beauty of nature and the changing seasons.

Nature suddenly bursting into flower is a great time to get outside and feel the joy. This activity invites you to create your own *Hanami* moment to facilitate soft fascination and experience the restorative benefits of nature. Attention Restoration Theory suggests that to do this we need to be free and feel immersed in the environment – away from everyday stressors. An ideal time would be during a break or after a busy day.

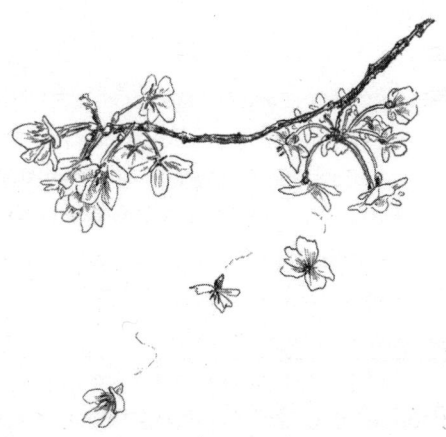

Search for a location where you feel comfortable and where there will be some blossom. You might need to plan ahead, noting the flower buds swelling in the weeks beforehand. Look for a place with a bench, log or spot on the grass by a tree in flower, such as a cherry or apple. Or perhaps near a hawthorn, with its distinctive foamy blossom. A place where you can sit comfortably and have a clear view of the flowers.

Take in the tree and let the sights, sounds and textures of nature around you capture your attention. Embrace the concept of soft fascination as you explore the blossom with your eyes, enjoying its beauty and fragility. Allow yourself to contemplate the transience of life and cherish this moment with the blooms, which will soon become petals delivered gently to the ground by the breeze.

## What we eat

If nature fits our senses and soothes our mind, what about our food? There are parallels between the natural stimuli that 'fit' our senses and whole foods that 'fit' our body and digestive system. Whole foods that are well-suited to our bodies and biological needs are easier to digest and provide nutrients that help us to function, bringing physical and mental health benefits. We feel better when our food is of the sort we have evolved to eat – a varied diet of roots, fruits, nuts, legumes and seeds. By contrast, the more processed and artificial foods we often eat now are having a negative impact on our health.

Just as it is good for us to be mindful and notice nature, we should try to be mindful and take more notice while we are eating, focusing on the taste, texture and aroma of what's in our mouth, and considering all the elements that contributed to creating that food, from sun and rain to harvesting and beyond.

People can find it easier to feel a connection to food than to nature. Perhaps unsurprisingly, nature connection tends to be stronger among those who live within a rural, farming environment. The distance between us and our food has grown. We no longer need to forage, and few people grow their own food. Most of us purchase it from supermarkets, where even whole foods such as vegetables arrive cleaned, processed and packaged. Our hunter-gatherer ancestors trusted nature to provide, while we now place our trust in supermarkets.

### *Activity*: Grow your own

Indoor salad growing is a simple way to start to bridge the gap between ourselves, our food and the natural world. It's an opportunity to step away from the convenience of the supermarket and reconnect with the natural processes that used to produce all our food. Growing salad leaves is possible in limited spaces like a windowsill, as long as the sunlight hits it for a few hours each day. Growing on a windowsill also enables you to witness up close the wonder of nature as seeds transform into edible plants. Here's how to get started.

#### *Gather your supplies*
For the novice, lettuces are excellent choices as they are relatively easy to grow. You'll need a tray, seeds and

potting compost (make sure it is peat-free). Ideally, your tray should have drainage holes, so you'll also need a tray for your tray! When choosing your seeds, opt for loose-leaf varieties like romaine lettuce or a mesclun mix. Another option are microgreens such as broccoli – young, edible greens that are harvested sooner, but disappear quickly.

*Sow the seeds and water*
Fill the tray with the potting compost. Sow the seeds according to the instructions on the packet. Moisten the soil.

*Care and harvesting*
Prod the soil every so often with your fingers to check whether it needs watering. Your aim is to keep it moist, but not soggy. As we'll see in October, this simple contact with the microbe-rich compost also contributes to our wellbeing. Cultivate a sense of wonder as you observe germination and the changes in your plants as they grow into seedlings and then, after a few weeks, develop leaves that are large enough to eat. Snip off the outer leaves, so that the inner leaves can continue growing. Celebrate your success as you wash them and taste them. Pay attention to the smell, texture and taste.

**Lost words**

Our disconnection from nature is reflected not just in

the increased distance between us and our food, but also in the decline of nature words in books and songs. Researchers have analysed how frequently nature words are used in works of fiction, songs and film scripts and have found a decline starting in the 1950s.[13]

Authors write about what matters to them, what is meaningful and what readers want to read. Language reflects culture and also shapes it. The decline in the use of words related to nature reflects its diminishing importance in people's lives, and this is likely to reduce further still. It shows that nature holds less significance for society.

While their worldviews are diverse, Indigenous peoples often have a close affinity with nature and this is reflected in their cultures. Work with Indigenous peoples has demonstrated that their connection to nature is not simply driven by repeated interaction with it; their stories and songs are themselves important pathways to a reciprocal relationship between them and the world around them. In your nature journal, try not just to describe and capture nature, but also to tell stories that convey its richness and significance. Meaning is a powerful pathway to deeper connections with nature; the written word is powerful too – and binding.

### *Activity*: Compile a nature playlist

Songs in particular can help create emotional connections that reignite our bond with nature. This activity involves compiling a nature playlist for the summer ahead, one that inspires you to explore and appreciate the natural world around you. Look for songs that contain lyrics that tap into the pathways to nature connection and celebrate nature. You might think folk music is the most obvious source, but consider a range of genres and see how far back in time you need to go. Write down the selected songs and artists in your journal and create a digital playlist. Enjoy them, but also take a moment to reflect on how the simple celebration of nature in song has decreased – what would you sing about?

Here are some of my favourites that are tuned into nature, the joy and wonder it brings, and that provide a reminder of the need to do more to care for it. All decades old, perhaps simpler times:

Nina Simone, 'Feeling Good' – 1965

Gil Scott-Heron, 'I Think I'll Call It Morning' – 1971

Minnie Riperton, 'Simple Things' – 1975

Louis Armstrong, 'What A Wonderful World' – 1967

Stevie Wonder, 'Summer Soft' – 1976

Marvin Gaye, 'Mercy Mercy Me (The Ecology)' – 1971

## Angel: The chiffchaff

April's angel is the chiffchaff. You probably heard its call in March, but the cheerful repeat of its song can fill the air in April. The chiffchaff is a small, sprightly bird that migrates to the UK each spring, heralding the awakening of nature and the vitality of the season. It holds a special place in the hearts of many nature enthusiasts.

The chiffchaff's distinctive, repetitive call echoes its name — 'chiff... chaff', as it rings through the woodlands. While its call is distinctive, the chiffchaff can be tricky to spot, especially as the trees come into leaf. Its plumage is mainly a muted olive green, although it has a paler belly and a darker eye stripe that provides another clue to its identity as it flits through branches.

After wintering in Africa, the chiffchaff embarks on an incredible journey to Europe for the bounty that spring brings. This migration is a reminder of the interconnectedness of ecosystems and the energy at the heart of all life.

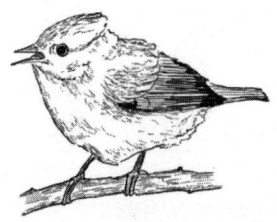

**For nature**: Do not disturb – people, pets and wildlife

The UK is a nation of pet lovers. Around 60% of households have a pet, up from 40% before the pandemic, which saw numbers increase by over 3 million. That's 12 million dogs and 12 million cats in 17 million homes. Unfortunately, being a nature lover and a pet lover can be a tricky combination.

Cat lovers know that it is natural for cats to hunt birds and mice. In the UK, it is thought that each year, cats kill over 200 million birds and mammals, plus some amphibians and reptiles.[14] It is difficult to verify such figures and they may seem extremely high, but across 12 million cats with a kill every two weeks or so on average, the total doesn't seem wildly unreasonable.

The effect of dogs is more subtle, but still significant. Most dog lovers do not think their dogs are a threat to wildlife. But to birds, dogs are a threat. When a dog is about, birds depart from their nests, leaving eggs unprotected from predators and cold air. Birds are disturbed by dogs, even when they are on leads. Research has found that dog walking can reduce woodland bird numbers by around 40%.[15] Beaches are a popular place for exercising a dog, but this presents several risks to shorebirds.[16] When a dog runs along the beach causing birds to take flight, it interrupts their feeding and forces them to expend precious energy. If this occurs repeatedly as other dog walkers pass, the waste of energy and loss of feeding time becomes significant – birds must feed many hours a day to survive. Dogs also eat chicks and crush the eggs of ground-nesting birds, with 50% of nests on a beach being trampled in one study.[17] There is no doubt that making beaches dog-free increases the number of birds. Of course, people disturb birds too.

Be aware of the impact you and your pet can have on nature. As you notice nature more, keep an eye out for birds and see if you can pass without causing them to take flight.

While we are on the subject of the impact of our pets on wildlife, a quick note on their food, and how this increases it further.[18] Figures vary, but producing the food required to feed the UK's cats and dogs is thought to release over 9 million tons of greenhouse gases each year – similar to the emissions from over 5 million SUV-type cars. Which makes the emissions from feeding the additional 3.2 million pandemic pets equivalent to some 750,000 SUVs on the road or burning half a million tonnes of coal a year. Pets are an important part of many people's lives. They provide companionship, meaningful relationships and entertainment – but so can connecting with nature, and without the ecological pawprint!

# MAY

How wonderful is the month of May? It's a magical time when spring bursts into its fullest and most glorious bloom. The days get warmer and longer still and everything responds: fresh leaves adorn once-bare trees, birds like the returning blackcap sing in chorus and countless flowers spring up in the meadows. Ferns fully unfurl, more butterflies appear and ponds are busy with tadpoles searching for food and hiding from predators. Verges, lanes and pathways are graced by waves of cow parsley, a cloud of white flowers that attract bees, hover-flies and butterflies – follow one on its trip from plant to plant. Traditional festivals celebrate this exuberance and can still be seen in customs such as Morris dancing, well dressings, maypoles and the crowning of the May Queen.

My nature journal notes from May reflect this vibrancy and diversity:

> *May sees Earth's flesh reform. Greens ooze*
> *from the darkness of the wood, as birdcalls*
> *pipe a therapeutic dose of life's spirit. About*
> *the wood the meadows deepen, blades curve*

*and take on a hint of the blue of the sky. The air itself thickens as I walk, warmed and nurtured like an organ in a greater body, beating a path speckled with blown petals from blossom. Such is the joy of May.*

## Forest bathing

Forest bathing, or *shinrin-yoku*, is a healing practice from Japan, in which people immerse themselves in woodland, pay attention to their senses and harmonise with nature. Forest bathing usually involves a walk in a forest, but it can also include exercises such as meditation, bushcraft, aromatherapy, cooking or yoga. From a research perspective, this can make identifying the exact factors needed for wellbeing and nature connection difficult, but overall there is evidence that *shinrin-yoku* can benefit mental wellbeing, for example increasing positive emotions, reducing rumination, anxiety and stress, and improving conditions such as depression.

Individual studies have also found a range of potential wider health benefits, from lowering blood pressure, improving cardiovascular health, boosting the immune system and reducing the stress hormone cortisol. It is thought that some of the benefits of forest bathing come through breathing in the natural organic compounds or phytoncides given off by the trees. They fill the air in the forest 'understorey' – the layer of trees and shrubs between the floor and the canopy – but are also found at low levels in other green spaces.

As you might expect, although not a primary aim, forest bathing also improves nature connection; in fact, this can be the largest benefit. The simple idea at the heart of forest bathing is to notice and appreciate nature. Noticing the various colours and patterns, watching movement, feeling the textures of bark, focusing on absorbing the aroma of leaves and the sounds of woodland.

### *Activity*: Forest, woodland or park bathing

Research suggests your forest-bathing session needs to be at least 20 minutes, but it can last an hour or two. Incidentally, despite the name, you don't have to go to a forest for this: studies have shown the benefits of forest bathing can be achieved in small bits of woodland and even among a cluster of trees in an urban park.

In a woodland or copse of trees, find a place to sit or recline with a view of another tree. Follow the trunk to a branch, and then another branch, exploring the twigs along the way. Wonder how a tree that stands stoutly divides itself to nothing, from its thick trunk, through slimmer branches, to just twigs and leaves. Notice the leaves, how they move with the breeze and filter the light. Look up into its own wilderness, a place untouched by human activity. Consider its life, its growth towards the light, the unfurling of its leaves, their fall. Consider the lives of the creatures in the tree.

Sit with the tree. Spend time with it.

When you're ready to, move on, look beneath the tree for leaves, noting the different colours as you wander. If you wish, smell the leaf litter from the woodland floor. Pause to listen and consider what you can hear, be it birds or the sound of the breeze. Approach a tree and explore it through touch alone. You can add your own activities from yoga to a picnic.

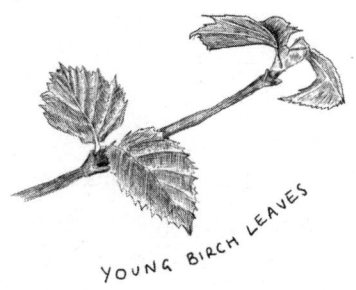

YOUNG BIRCH LEAVES

## How nature manages our moods

The surprising thing about forest-bathing research is that much of the work didn't consider emotions – or at least the significant role it plays in regulating our emotions and managing our moods. To better understand the role nature plays in our well being, it's important to understand that emotions are much more than feelings that emerge every now and again. They are fundamental aspects of human function, involving our nervous system, heart and brain. As different emotions come and go, they shape our actions and responses to everyday demands, so regulating them is vital for us to function optimally.

A useful framework for understanding emotional regulation and its influence on mental well being is the three-circle model of emotion regulation devised by Professor Paul Gilbert.[19] As a model, it is a simplification of very complex physiological processes, offering an accessible way to understand how the natural world helps manage our moods.

The three dimensions of our emotion regulation system are drive, contentment and threat:

1. *Drive* represents positive feelings that motivate us to seek out resources and achieve success. It also encompasses the joy and pleasure we experience as we pursue our goals.
2. *Contentment* covers affiliation, togetherness and positive feelings of affection, soothing and kindness. It represents a calm with the way things are – once the pursuit of goals has been achieved, perhaps.
3. *Threat* encompasses the anxious feelings and alerts generated by our threat and self-protection system. This system, located in the fast-acting amygdala, can be both activating and inhibiting.

I explain this model by using natural symbols to represent the three core types of emotions. So, for drive, imagine a swift, its rapid flight as it hunts for food, bringing us joy; for contentment, imagine a blackbird, its song a soothing presence; and for anxiety, imagine a thistle, its thorns representing angst and unease.

Each of these three dimensions bring different feelings, motivations and behaviours. And achieving wellbeing requires maintaining a balance between them. When one dimension is overactive, such as when we are overly driven, it can disrupt the balance and reduce positive emotions, leaving room for anxiety to take hold. Over time this can develop into conditions like depression.

When people are monitored resting either in natural or urban areas, we've found their responses fit the model of drive, contentment and threat. Unsurprisingly, being in nature was mainly found to be calming (symbolised by the song of the blackbird), activating the parasympathetic nervous system, which is associated with contentment. On the other hand, being in an urban environment tended to stimulate the sympathetic nervous system, which is associated with drive and threat (the swift and thistle). This is represented by the arc of emotion in the illustration below – imagine a needle swinging across the arc, with nature engagement drawing it away from threat and anxiety.

However, the story was more nuanced. Some people found being in nature stimulating, while others felt anxious about what might be lurking in the undergrowth. This would cause an increase in sympathetic nervous system activity, swinging the needle towards the thistle. On the other hand, those more attuned to nature felt exhilaration when spending time in the woods, causing the needle to settle on the swift. This research shows how nature plays a crucial role in helping balance our emotions in the short-term and also highlights the interconnection between us and the rest of nature.

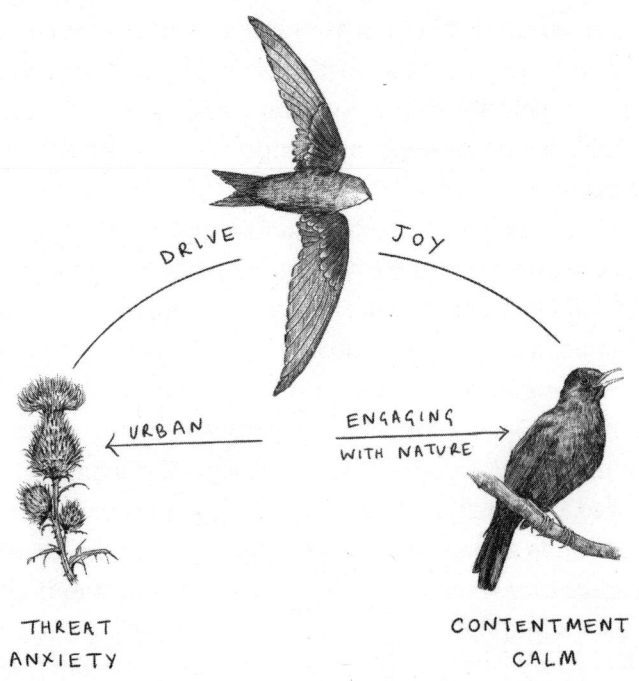

DRIVE

JOY

← URBAN

ENGAGING
WITH NATURE →

THREAT
ANXIETY

CONTENTMENT
CALM

## Reflection

May is a great month to find joy and calm. It is a month when the warmer weather motivates us to get outside more and plan trips into nature. So why not use the process of planning to boost your connection with nature before you leave? Reflecting on where you are going to go, and what form your trip is going to take, can create a closer relationship with nature. As we saw with the awe walk, sometimes a simple prompt can make a real difference. But while awe is a passing emotion, meaning has a longer-term effect on our well-being, what is important to us and feels worthwhile. Reflecting for a few minutes on why that is has been found to be beneficial.[20]

### *Activity*: Reflecting on nature

For this activity, you can spend a few minutes with your nature journal. Consider how nature influences your planning and the role it plays. Imagine your planned visit to a beautiful spot in nature. Think about the things you will do and ask yourself which parts of nature would bring most meaning, and why. For example, you might plan a trip to a favourite viewpoint, a place where the landscape makes you feel part of a larger whole. Or to a woodland glade where the rich variety of sights and sounds weave you into the wider life force.

### Mindful attention

While reflection involves thought and valuing the past or future, mindfulness is the practice of deliberately paying attention to the present moment. Being mindful involves developing a heightened sense of awareness of one's body, thoughts, emotions and the surrounding environment in an accepting and non-judgemental way. It includes observing thoughts as passing events rather than as essential representations of who we are. Allowing thoughts to come and go without expanding and reflecting on them helps with focusing on the present moment in nature. Mindfulness revolves around noticing what is taking place rather than thinking about it. It can bring emotional balance and wellbeing and it has been found to enhance the impact of experience in nature, and thereby to strengthen nature connection.

When comparing reflection and mindful attention in our research, we found reflection on emotions, values and the self better explained higher levels of nature connection. However, there's a good amount of evidence that mindfulness, experiencing nature in the moment, can increase nature connection. The good news is that one approach doesn't need to replace the other. Those moments of enhanced experience of nature can be the basis of later reflection. And everyone is different. Some may find reflection works well for them, while others might prefer mindfulness.

### *Activity*: Mindful connection with birdsong

This activity is an invitation simply to engage with bird-song in a mindful and present way. It also helps develop the skill of noticing when your attention wanders. The basic principles can be applied to other aspects of nature connection until it becomes habitual.

*Prepare*

- Find a quiet, comfortable and peaceful space outside or near an open window where you can sit comfortably and hear birds.
- Adopt a posture that allows you to be relaxed yet alert. You can stand or walk if that works better for you.
- Tune into your breath: take a few slow, deep breaths, noticing the sensation of each inhalation and exhalation. Allow your breath to deepen, let go of any tension or distractions and settle into the present moment.

*Listen*

- Listen attentively and shift your focus to the birdsong. Listen openly without judgement or reflection.
- Notice the variety of sounds, different melodies and rhythms, and the spaces in between.
- Stay present within the sounds; the birdsong is your anchor. If your attention or thoughts wander, gently refocus on the birdsong.
- Choose one call that captures your attention. Follow it through the air, noting its variety of tone, its rise and fall. Be absorbed by a single melody.

- Let your awareness expand, broaden your listening to the entire soundscape, buzzing insects, rustling leaves. Notice how they blend and weave together.
- As you listen, appreciate the gift of birdsong, the sounds of nature. Develop a sense of gratitude and recognise the interconnectedness of all living beings.
- Be receptive to your other senses: the sensations in your body, the warmth of the sun on your skin or the feeling of the breeze.
- Remain open to the experience of the present moment and allow yourself to be immersed in the sounds for as long as you feel comfortable, fully present and engaged.
- When you are ready to finish, gently bring your attention back to your own breath and calmly transition back to the everyday.

*Repeat, adapt and reflect*

- Practise your mindful moments regularly, perhaps ten minutes each day, to build a deeper connection with nature. Simply spending time in nature has been found to increase mindfulness. Remember, you can adapt the instructions to fit your preferences and circumstances. You can also explore other spaces and add variation; for example, try walking instead of sitting.
- Also, consider journalling about your experience. What did you notice about the character of

the birdsong? How did it affect your emotions? Did you gain any insights from this mindful connection with nature?

- Finally, you can adapt this practice to focus on other elements of nature, for example water. Consider the ripples from rain in a puddle or sit by a river watching the eddies come and go.

## Angel: The swallow

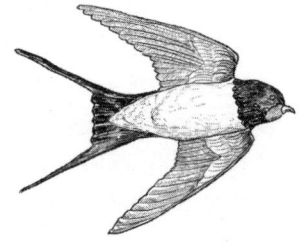

A notable bird of May is the swallow. Each year, swallows complete an amazing journey of thousands of miles, navigating their way from Africa, across the Sahara Desert and Mediterranean Sea to reach the UK. It takes them several weeks. One can imagine the challenges presented by the distance, the weather, navigation, predators and the availability of food. Such a journey for a small bird is incredible and something to reflect on and celebrate with every swallow you see. With their dark-blue and glossy backs, red throats and pair of long tail feathers, they are easy to spot as they chase the midges and gnats that populate the May air or weave their way above the fields. These agile fliers can be found in open farmland, parks and close to water, their call a chattering cascade of notes like falling beads. I enjoy following their flight patterns in the air. A summer angel.

### *For nature*: Rest your mower and liberate a lawn

The UK has lost 97% of its flower-rich meadows since the 1970s, and that loss has had a significant impact on wildlife. One easy way we can all help to reverse this sad trend is to give our mowers a rest and let our lawns grow wild. There are millions of lawns across the UK that could be turned into flower-rich grassy areas, and indeed much is already being done to promote the idea (for example, No Mow May, an annual campaign by the conservation charity Plantlife).

If you don't want to lose your whole lawn, just give up a patch of it. Personally, I enjoy mowing curving pathways across the lawn and wandering along them to see what emerges. The paths also make the lawn look quite 'neat' and cared for, if that's a concern for you. If you don't have a lawn, consider encouraging your workplace or local authority to reduce the mowing of verges and parks.

Letting lawns bloom with wildflowers provides valuable sources of food for pollinators like bees and butterflies. It also helps create a little more biodiversity

– which means more nature to notice.

Plantlife offers guidance and resources to help people take part. This includes a guide to liberating your lawn and managing the transition from mown to wild. There are also materials to help spread awareness of the campaign.

# JUNE

June sees the start of summer, full of youthful zest. Hedgerows and meadows are vivid, their sweet fragrance carried by the air. Sunlight plays on leafy canopies and shady woodlands are alive with unfurled ferns and unique scents. Birds are busy feeding their fledglings, and blackbirds are approaching their final month of song. Insects hover from flower to flower, gathering nectar and pollen. Dragonflies zip along the waterways, another thread in the ecosystem we are part of. The days are long, and the evenings can be warm, making it easy to find time to explore nature's many gifts. By the coast, pathways are bordered by wildflowers with sparkling seas beyond. Seabirds bring high-rise life to rocky cliffs and swoop along the shoreline, looking for food

My own nature journal notes reflect the joys and meaning of a June day to me:

> *Greenfinches called of lazy summer days and the rain of the summer so far was forgotten. Under a closing sky, a blackbird told of its day and year, for soon it would sing no more. The sky moved slowly, trying to halt time so*

*the blackbird's song would never end, part of it darkening and then taking on the bird's form, before returning to drifting cloud. I felt that the sky, indeed the evening itself, was a feather against a globe. And that globe was an eye within a bird.*

## Flower power

We've now seen how our physical and mental health can benefit from engaging with nature, whether from total immersion in it or simply noticing a few good things each day. And how the soft fascination of nature provides restoration and bathing in woodland brings yet more benefits. The diversity of the natural world is so immense that our possible connections to it are practically limitless. How important is it to experience a range of connections? Can a single element of nature be the basis of connection and wellbeing? Might viewing a single flower have a positive impact on our bodies?

Laboratory research has investigated the effect of viewing a single flower on blood pressure and stress.[21] In fact, it was not even a real flower; it was a photograph of a white chrysanthemum, with no stem or leaves. For only six seconds. Those taking part in this study were first shown a 'stress' image, something negative, or violent. Then they viewed either the flower or one of a variety of other images: a mosaic of pixels (similar to a QR code), a fixation point (a plus symbol), a picture of the sky or a chair, while their blood pressure was continuously monitored. The researchers found that their blood pressure decreased significantly more when participants had viewed the flower than when they'd viewed the other images.' However, interestingly, when the participants were asked to rate the level of their positivity after each image, they reported that both the sky and the flower turned their emotions back from negative to positive, with the sky rating higher even though it actually had less impact on the body. Either way, the study showed that natural elements bring calm.

The reason the flower affected the body in this way can again be explained by the soft fascination of nature, which readily holds our attention, freeing us from unpleasant thoughts and feelings. In a second study on the effect of viewing a flower, the research team measured the levels of cortisol – a hormone that helps the body manage stress – in the participants' saliva. And just as it lowered the participants' blood pressure in the first experiment, viewing a single flower, this time for eight minutes, was found to reduce their cortisol levels. Simply viewing a flower affects the systems of the body. Amazing!

A third element of the same research, in which the scientists used functional magnetic resonance imaging to explore brain activity, revealed that viewing the flower produced brain activation patterns associated with emotion regulation, which explains the reduction of the negative feelings induced by viewing the unpleasant images. Activation of the amygdala, linked to our fight or flight response, decreased. Similar decreases in activity were found in emotion-processing parts of the hippocampus, thereby suppressing negative memories

The conclusion was that the act of viewing a flower decreases negative emotion and accelerates the recovery of the body's stress response. It reduces the sympathetic nervous system activity linked to threat, as described by the arc of emotion that we looked at last month. That the image of a flower can automatically have an impact on the brain, nervous and hormone system in this way is a fascinating sign of the deep hidden connections we retain with nature. We are hard-wired to be calmed by nature, like a child in a parent's embrace.

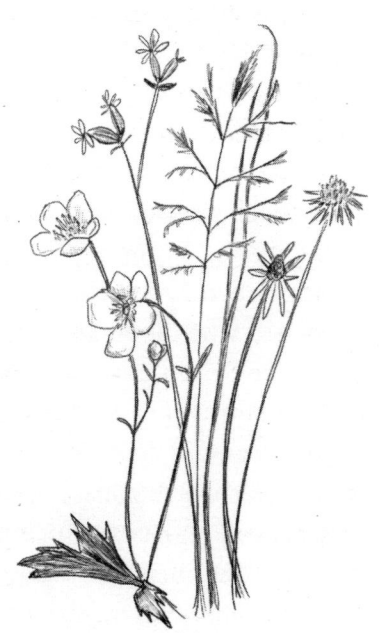

Humans evolved from primates in natural environments over 6–7 million years. According to this timescale, the rapid growth in urbanisation since the Industrial Revolution – a key point in our disconnection from nature – amounts to less than 0.01% of our history. In recent decades, with our immersion in artificial environments, this disconnection has increased markedly, further contributing to our stressed state. Arguably, we are not yet attuned to our new environment. Going 'back to nature' returns our bodies to their natural state.

Modern science is revealing how our bodies respond to flowers, yet they have had deep meaning forus for many centuries. Back in June 2012, when I was midway through writing my way to nature connection, I was walking by the River Trent with my eight-year-old daughter when she spotted the pale, pink-tinged petals of a wild rose lying on the path before us. 'I wonder why they are heart-shaped?' she asked. It was only then that I realised the rose petal was indeed a perfect heart shape. Assuming this must be the origin of the heart-shaped symbol so ubiquitous in our lives, I was surprised when I researched it later to find there was no reference to it. Given that the rose has been a symbol of love since Roman times at least, and the wild rose is native across Asia, Europe and North America, the idea seems worth consideration – and is certainly more compelling and beautiful than Freud's theory of the heart symbol being based on various parts of human anatomy. But then Sigmund Freud was no nature lover, writing about humans, as he did, coming together and 'taking up the attack on nature, thus forcing it to obey human will, under the guidance of science'.[22] The culture of disconnection and dominion over nature is now deeply embedded, yet it can be deconstructed by a single flower.

*Activity*: **Find a flower**

Let's put the science into practice in the simplest of ways. Find a flower and look at it for a few minutes. Ideally, it will be a pollinator-friendly bloom you've grown – perhaps one that's emerged in the unmown grass from May. Exploring the micro-world within a lawn can be fascinating, with the tiniest of flowers hidden away. Whatever you've chosen, view it as you wish, openly and in the moment, or think about how the photons of light reflected on such a delicate organism can change the physiology of the body in seconds.

You may like to consider whether different flowers mean different things to you. Many wildflowers have historical meanings, representing specific emotions or myths, legends and traditions. Some wildflowers can evoke a sense of identity, representing the lands where they bloom, for example. You may also have your own personal meanings, a daisy returning you to a playing field or picnic. Which flower would you choose to represent you?

## Solstice and spirituality

Humans search for meaning, and nature often evokes a sense of belonging to something larger than oneself. Each June, thousands of people gather at Stonehenge to celebrate the summer solstice. For many of us, the solstice provides a rare moment when we become aware of the movements of the sun and ancient traditions such as Druidism. For our ancestors, the movements of the sun and changing seasons were critical to their existence, and this fed through to their belief system.

Over 4000 years ago, people in the west of Britain embarked on a huge effort to gather, transport and align hefty rocks with the movements of the sun. The stones of Stonehenge frame the rising sun on the longest day of the year and the setting sun on the shortest day of the year. Ancient peoples will have gathered to witness – and probably celebrate – these pivotal moments. These traditions faded many centuries ago, but the alignment of Stonehenge with the sun was 'rediscovered' in the 1700s, and last century, there was a revival in the spiritual significance of the structure, as well as of pagan beliefs, with thousands gathering for the solstice.

Pagan was a term often used to refer to non-Christians, but modern paganism covers a broad spectrum of spiritual beliefs and ways of expressing spiritual relationships, including Druidism. Historically, Druids were religious leaders in ancient Celtic cultures, but the modern Druid movement evolved from a mix of liberal Christian traditions, some fragments of Celtic tradition and nature worship. Although the movement is very varied, most Druids believe in the divine essence of nature and promote a harmonious relationship with both its physical and spiritual aspects. Aspects such as flow, wholeness, beauty are among core values. Nature is divine and is the source of the symbols and imagery of Druid myth and practice.

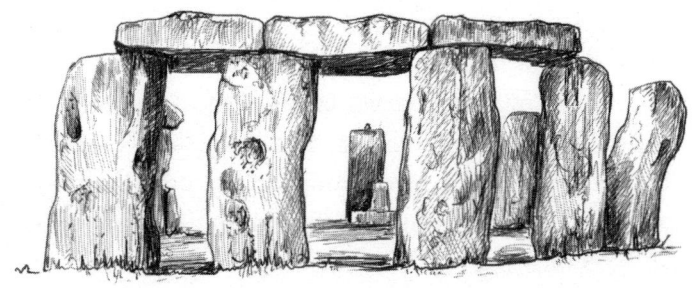

For some, such beliefs and celebrations may seem esoteric or eccentric, yet the Christian holiday of the feast of Saint John the Baptist also celebrates the summer solstice, as does the Midsummer festival in Sweden. Our spiritual needs are expressed in many forms, with spirituality referring to the deepest values that guide us, our inner beliefs and personal experiences. Spirituality is a complex, abstract, subjective search for meaning and transcendence beyond the present. It can involve sacredness, and harmony with some higher power. Whether it be in an organised religion, or in a passion for nature or a football team, people find meaning and belonging in many ways. Spirituality is universally experienced and transcends religion.

Given that spirituality is associated with lasting and meaningful wellbeing, we should not be surprised to learn that there is a body of research into its link with nature connectedness – not a large amount, but still worth noting. Awe-inspiring views of nature have been found to increase feelings of spirituality; and correspondingly, people with a closer bond with nature tend to have a greater spiritual orientation. This makes sense, as nature connection is a bond with a world beyond the human one, an expansion of *self* to include all life forms. Research has shown that the deeper wellbeing that comes from nature connection is derived in part from the spiritual fulfilment that we achieve by having a close relationship with nature; a spiritual interconnectedness links us to the wider natural world.

At a time of ever-increasing individualism in Western society, with so much emphasis on 'I' and 'me', this connection is key, as an excessive preoccupation with the self is a growing barrier to pro-nature behaviours. As we saw in April, an important feature of many Indigenous cultures is a strong spiritual connection with nature. Compare this to our Western bias, which tends to focus on how nature will benefit *us*.

Many of us may happily concur with the idea of the natural world and ecosystems of the Earth being 'sacred', but zoom into the constituent parts, ask yourself: are forests and woodlands sacred? Is a tree sacred? The Sycamore Gap tree felled in Northumberland in

2023 seemed to hold a special place in people's hearts, and the felling of urban trees can cause wide consternation. But what about a leaf, the caterpillar upon it, or the beetle within its bark? Does our appreciation of the sacredness of our planet's ecosystem that gives us all life have a limit? For the people of Meghalaya in India, cutting twigs and flowers from sacred forests would be offensive to their deities. The degradation of these forests is linked to the erosion of traditional values. Most communities in the Western world have a religious sacred site, a church or mosque, for example. How many communities have a place where nature is sacred?

There have been many studies into spirituality and wilderness experiences in Western cultures. There's little wilderness left in the UK, but week-long expeditions to remote areas of Scotland have been found to increase nature connection. Such expeditions typically involve total nature immersion with no access to mobile phones, electricity or even running water, and include a range of activities from wild swimming and foraging to canoeing and nature watching. It's worth noting that the more 'outward-bound', adventure-focused expeditions tend not to lead to increases in nature connection. Individual exploration is more likely to bring us closer to nature than a prescriptive challenge.

We have covered considerable ground here, from the summer solstice at Stonehenge, through Druidism and the importance of spirituality in general to the spiritual aspects of nature connection and wilderness. Preparing for a week of total nature immersion would take a book of its own. So, the next activity returns to the summer solstice, but before we do that, why not take a moment to reflect on your typical holidays and trips? You may already be a keen camper; if not, think about how your next trip might take a step towards being off-grid and immersed in nature, remembering it doesn't need to be an outward-bound challenge!

### *Activity*: Celebrate the summer solstice

This activity is to celebrate the longest day of the year, the high point of summer. You might consider starting your own tradition, one that could grow in your community. Take some time to plan your summer solstice celebration, always remembering that at its heart should be the principle of being in harmony with nature. Your celebration might reflect the values and beliefs that guide you. It might contain certain elements of nature, a simple offering, take you beyond the present or simply be an off-grid gathering in nature, perhaps in a place that feels sacred to you, your family, friends or community – and where you can share stories with a nature theme.

It could take place at sunrise, or sunset. It could include a walk to a hilltop, seasonal whole food or sitting peacefully in the light of the setting sun as you write your annual solstice poem and wait for the stars to appear. Whatever is meaningful.

## Angel: The starling

June's angel is the starling, a star that can be enjoyed in many unlikely places. From afar, the starling can appear dark and plain, yet close up its feathers are iridescent and its sleek form shimmers with emerald and purple. Once somewhat maligned when it used to descend into gardens in large numbers, the starling is more likely these days to be spotted in city squares or busy harbours. Where humans gather, starlings tend to gather too, bringing a cheerful chatter, mischievous antics and their own community. As starling numbers have declined, it has become more appreciated, a reminder that nature's beauty and wonder can be found in the busiest of locations. Its charm brings magic to our greyest spaces.

## *Activity*: Get to know a tree

Back in January, you found a local tree to get to know month by month. In March, you returned to track the spring awakening of your tree and witness its buds emerging. It is now June, and you will have seen your tree transform to be fully dressed, its fresh leaves full of zest and harbouring summer sunshine. Insects may gather around it too. Spend a moment with your tree, trace its form once more. Watch the play of sunlight through the branches, the shadow of leaves patterning the trunk. Perhaps you can shelter from a passing shower or enjoy the shade from the midday sun, a calm summer retreat.

### *For nature*: Create homes for insects

Insects are often overlooked, or considered a source of irritation or even fear, but they are a critical part of the ecosystem. And they can be surprisingly rewarding and entertaining to watch, with their diversity of intricate forms and busy explorations. So, there's great value in creating homes for insects. The best way to do this, of course, is to let nature provide a home through wild-life-friendly gardening. But if you don't have a garden, or the space for this, here are a few simple suggestions for how to make a bug hotel – no measuring or straight lines needed.

Many shop-bought bug hotels look nice but they don't provide great homes for wildlife. They are often too small and don't have enough entrances: a good bug hotel should be accessible from at least three sides. Bee hotels should be stable rather than left to hang in the wind, and their entry holes should be the correct size: not too big and not too shallow.

In a spare box or even a bit of discarded wooden furniture, assemble unwanted items, such as bricks with air holes, offcuts of wood, broken terracotta pots, fallen twigs and branches and dried leaves. If your container is big and sturdy enough, you can stack it with offcuts of wood, or create shelves with bricks in between, and then stuff twigs, dried leaves and broken pots into the shelves. You're basically looking to create some nooks and crannies to provide a place of safety. Whatever you do, use natural materials, avoiding treated wood or plastics. You can even give it a green sedum roof! When your creation is complete, place your hotel in a sheltered spot away from people, direct sunlight and strong winds. It makes sense to raise it off the soil on a spare slab or a few bricks. Insects like spiders, beetles, woodlice and ladybirds will hopefully move in.

As their name suggests, it's best for solitary bees to have their own hotel, as spiders can eat them. Solitary bees like to nest in tubes. One popular method to create a home for them is to bundle short lengths of hollow bamboo cane – these should be 15cm long with natural holes of between 2 and 12mm in diameter, clean and splinter-free. As with birdfeeders, it's recommended that you clean and refresh the bee hotel each spring after any young have hatched.

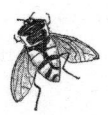

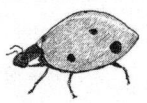

# JULY

July is the middle of summer, offering a hopeful prospect of hours of unbroken sunshine illuminating flowers in bloom, busy bumblebees and swifts soaring above. Many young birds will have fully fledged by now, and a host of insects will be joining them in flight. Ponds and lakes glisten, and we might seek the cool air of a woodland or the coast. Yet July is the time in nature's calendar when the new blooms start to decrease and the signs of fruiting start to show. It's a month to savour, a turning point when the blackbirds fall silent – make sure to listen out for their final boast of summer; let their song be a twine for your thoughts to climb as you anticipate the summer months ahead.

My nature journal notes reflect the meaning of July:

> *I sought refuge from a July shower in the woods, finding a pool of darkness, reflected trunks sinking into a deep pit with shafts of light. The blackbird shared the woodland darkness, its alarm call stitched across the gloom like a beak orange thread. The rain passed and I was able to walk the familiar*

*landscape by the River Dove, the sun as
constant as the river. Dragonflies hovered
above it, their whirring mechanical flight
described wires in the air as a yellow-
hammer passed. I let an alder be the centre
of my gaze as I moved, trying to garner as
much as possible about its reality. The sky
extended longer than the land, curving and
capping the landscape, a backdrop to the
swifts however high they flew. I heard the
river over the wind in the shallows and as I
stood in the heat, five chasing swifts became
twelve, rising until their blades sliced the
sky's limits, fragments of sound falling like
sparks from punctures that would become
stars.*

## The impact of technology

We are nothing without technology. It defines humans
to the extent that few, if any of us, could survive from
nature alone. We can turn to technology for all of
our needs. Only the air that we breathe hasn't been
commodified. While nature sustains the other great
apes, the role of the natural world in our lives is
becoming ever more distant.

In April we saw how the use of nature words in books,
films and songs has declined, showing that nature holds
less meaning in our lives. The research on this decline

also considered why, and found that, rather than being linked to urbanisation, it was the dawn of new technology that most likely accounted for it. Television, video games, the internet and smartphones are the new technologies that shape our lives.

Smartphones are an interesting example. Widespread and ever present, they have put a vast range of functionality into our pockets. Our studies have found that higher levels of smartphone adoption are linked to lower levels of individual nature connection. Selfie-taking is edging nature out of the way. We also found that people with a stronger connection with nature take fewer pictures of themselves and more of nature. However, we can't demonise technology: we're technological apes! We need to include technology and smartphones within a new relationship with nature. It's not the tool that is to blame, after all; it's the use we put it to: a simple pen can be used to write a poem about a tree or sign a contract to cut down a forest.

And technology *can* be a tool for nature connection. Researchers have found that, when asked to take photographs of the things in nature that evoked emotions in them for a period of two weeks, people experienced significantly higher levels of nature connection compared to those who did the same with buildings, objects and the like.[23] And the benefits didn't stop there: those in the nature photography group experienced more positive feelings, and a greater sense of connection to other people and pro-social orientation, to give the formal term, than those in the other groups. A key thing in this work was that those taking part didn't spend any more time in nature; they were simply encouraged to notice it more and to be more aware of their emotions, such as hope, peace and awe.

In another study, people were asked to use their smartphones to photograph, video or record the sounds of beautiful things in nature.[24] Just one short walk led to increases in nature connection, with those taking part feeling happy, peaceful, calm and relaxed.

Hopefully you have fond memories of your awe walk in March. Better still, perhaps finding wonder and awe in everyday nature is now the norm for you. The study into the benefits of awe walks also included a photography task, with participants being asked to record the impact of their walks by taking a picture of themselves before, during, and after it.[25] Analysis of over 1000 photos led to some fascinating findings. Firstly, they looked at smile intensity and found that this increased during the walk in comparison to the control group. Secondly, they looked at the size of the person in proportion to the whole photo to measure 'self-size'. Those on awe walks tended to make themselves smaller and less prominent in the photo: there was more nature and a smaller self. Experiencing awe can shift how people view themselves, diverting attention from the self onto the vastness of the wilder world. This 'smallness' encourages us to see ourselves as part of something bigger, reducing our ego and promoting feelings of humility and kindness to others – a key element of wisdom.

The way we live today has created a culture of duality

and division – us and them, us and nature. But as we've seen, through re-engaging with nature, noticing its beauty, finding an emotional bond and meaning, we can break down these imagined boundaries. A term for this is 'ego dissolution'. I certainly found that reconnecting with nature changed my understanding of my *self* and my shared place within the wider natural world.

Interestingly, research has found that people taking LSD report a similar form of ego dissolution.[26] Scans have demonstrated that certain parts of the brain become more connected, increasing communication between areas associated with self-consciousness and sensory areas and thereby forming a stronger link between the self and the environment. This explains some of the science, but we don't need LSD for nature connection; we can take a trip into nature armed just with pen and journal or smartphone, and our sense of awe.

### *Activity*: A trip into nature

This activity invites you to use the technology that can separate you from nature to grow your connection, by using your smartphone's camera as a portal to explore wonders hidden in plain sight. Let's take it step by step.

*Step 1: Find a nature spot and stop*
Start with a little nature on a sunny day, be it your backyard, balcony or a quiet corner of your local

park; the kind of day when it's too warm to do much else. Sit, lie or wander around in search of a bit of natural beauty or something that evokes an emotion: a flower emerging from a crack in the pavement, the veins of a leaf or the bark of a tree.

### Step 2: Capture the feeling of beauty

Reach for your phone; take your time to slow down and to consider your subject, the viewpoint and how it appears on screen as you explore the options. Then take your photo, avoiding a flurry of clicks. Make a note of the feelings that drew you to take this photo.

### Step 3: Unleash other dimensions

Try experimenting with your phone's built-in features to move beyond a basic snapshot to an image, video or audio recording that amplifies the beauty you see and emotion you feel. You can:

- use the slow-motion feature to slow down the movements of a flower in the breeze or a bee on the wing. This can be a little tricky, but is worth pursuing: one second of success can provide several seconds of awe.
- speed up the passing of the day. Condense the movement of clouds or blooming flower into a few seconds using the timelapse feature. Then marvel at the clouds crossing the sky, or the setting sun sinking down below the horizon.
- get closer. See how close you can go before your

camera loses focus. Can you capture a drop of rain clinging to a twig, the texture of moss on a stone, or the delicate patterns within the wilderness of a single flower?

*Step 4: Pause, reflect and share*
Find a shady spot and go through what you've captured. Reflect on your choices, what caught you in the moment and the new insights from slowing down the passing of time. Jot your thoughts down in your journal and consider using technology to share your favourite moments on social media, perhaps inspiring others to turn tech from a tool of disconnection into one of discovery.

## The impact of becoming urban

Although technology is a major cause of our disconnection with nature, urbanisation is a factor too, as mentioned earlier. During the Industrial Revolution, people increasingly left their rural lives to work in factories and within a generation experienced an extinction of nature engagement. Progress was driven by the industrial exploitation of natural resources. More and more trees were felled, not just for shipbuilding but also to erect pit props as coal fuelled the human desire to conquer and break free from the bonds of nature. A perceived right to exploit nature took hold.

Unsurprisingly, countries with more urban dwellers

tend to have a weaker relationship with nature. Researchers have found that urban dwellers have a limited understanding of the intricate interdependence between humans and nature. They typically spend just five minutes a day in a green space, and are more likely to gaze at buildings than nature. The capacity to attend to and explore natural views is diminished. The natural world falls mute. Yet our perceptual systems prefer nature to artificial stimuli. Our minds are receptive to the views and sounds of the natural world. Nature is the gift we evolved to receive. And the good news is that it is possible to enjoy the sustained benefits of nature connection and mental wellbeing in urban environments. We just need a prompt.

Our research team developed a smartphone app that prompted users to notice the good things in nature when they were near an urban green space. After just one week of using it, there were significant improvements in nature connection and mental wellbeing – and these persisted for a month.

A handy aspect of this research was that we could see what the good things in urban nature were. A key source of wonder was encountering everyday wildlife, simple creatures we might find in a park, squirrels chasing each other, or bird song. Then came trees, followed by skies – both easy to find in an urban environment. People also valued greenery planted in built-up spaces, flowering plants and water, though less so.

## *Activity*: Go on an urban nature safari

Most of us live in residential areas surrounded by build-ings, if not in a town or city. These places offer many opportunities to go on an urban safari and seek out nature.

- Choose your urban wilderness. This could be a green space, a park or a churchyard, but you could also challenge yourself and head for a built-up area to see how nature is finding a way.
- Select your focus. You might decide to go in search of sensory experiences, emotional encounters, meaningful moments or nature's beauty. Or to see specific things, such as animals, birds or trees. Or sights, sounds and textures.
- Gather your tools. Download maps or nature identification guides. Maybe take a pair of binoc-ulars or even a magnifying glass.
- Head out when you have plenty of time to spare, and as ever, slow down!
- Explore your chosen location, seeking out as many types of moments as possible.
- Add your safari to your nature journal.

## Blue spaces

The vast majority of people in the UK do not live within easy reach of the coast. But many of us can visit inland lakes and waterways instead, and it is well worth trying to do so. Clearly, hills, trees and meadows are wonderful features, but the 'blue spaces' of beaches, lakes and rivers offer something green alone cannot.

Living near greener landscapes is good for you, but living near the coast or near a lake is linked to even better mental health, particularly if you have a view of the water. Weekly visits to blue spaces have also been found to be beneficial, and can potentially help people with anxiety. Specific 'blue care' or 'blue space interventions' have been shown to deliver improved mental health, as have water sport activities like surfing, kayaking and scuba diving.

Open, freshwater swimming has become very fashionable in recent years, with people often describing the experience as not just emotional but spiritual, prompting feelings of being part of something greater than oneself. Wild swimming, in particular, has been linked to a range of mental health benefits and even some evidence of enhanced immune function.

Clearly, swimming is an immersive experience, and doing it in a wild environment where sensations and interactions with nature are brought to the fore, can stimulate a deep sense of connectedness and potential reorientation of perspective. It is important to point out that wild swimming should be undertaken with care and precaution, as the cold water can have a powerful impact on the body – starting out with a club is highly advisable.

For those who don't like the water, remember that

land-based activities near the coast are good for us too! Walking is still a great option – and much easier to fit into one's daily life than scuba diving.

### *Activity*: **Paddling on the shoreline**

July is an ideal month for visiting the coast and this activity is something we can all still enjoy when we're there. It's a time to revisit your childhood (equipped with the knowledge introduced in this book).

Go barefoot on the beach. Embrace the simplicity of a paddle along the shore. Focus on the sensations, the cold of the water as you wade, the change with each step. Feel the sand that resists like bone and then gives like flesh. Listen to the rhythm of the sea, the beat of breaking waves, the cries of gulls and breathe in the salty air deeply.

Scan the shoreline for nature's gifts – seashells, pebbles, seaweed and feathers – the many shapes and colours that speak of the ocean's diversity of life. Do some appeal more than others? Do they prompt a sense of wonder or curiosity?

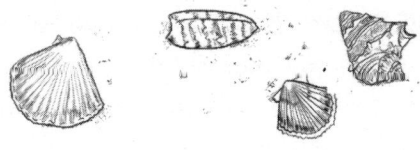

Pause by any rockpools to search for hidden wonders. Perhaps arrange a few shells, pebbles or seaweed to create a pattern. Imagine the journeys these objects have been on to share this moment with you. Above all embrace the simple joy of the coast as you splash through the shallows.

## Angel: The swift

Swifts are very remarkable birds, specially adapted to life on the wing. Their narrow, curved wings and forked tails make them the fastest birds in level flight, and also allow agility at speed as they chase insects and drink by skimming the surface of lakes. In addition to being fast, they fly vast distances, having one of the longest migrations to and from Africa. Swifts nesting in colonies about our buildings are a real highlight of any urban safari. Learn to recognise their distinctive screeching calls and you will be ready to catch their display. Groups of swifts often bring drama to our streets as they wheel and turn close to rooftops, their feathered blades flashing in the evening sun, cutting our thoughts free to float with them in azure skies. Before they start to leave at the end of July, find a place to sit back and watch their antics: a garden in an urban pub can be ideal!

### *For nature*: Take part in a butterfly count

Citizen science can be a great way of bringing us into harmony with nature, increasing wellbeing and pro-nature action. There are many projects that involve counting insects and butterflies. Our research has found that the benefits of these activities can be enhanced if we also try to notice the good things in nature as we count. This in turn makes us more likely to want to do more for nature. The Big Butterfly Count is a UK mass-participation citizen science project that gathers data on the abundance of a range of butterfly and moth species. It is run by Butterfly Conservation and usually runs over a few weeks from mid-July. It simply involves counting the number and type of butterflies you see. Taking part is straightforward:

> *Step 1*: Get ready, download the ID chart or smartphone app.
> *Step 2*: Join in by choosing a place to spot butterflies and moths for 15 minutes. Record what you see and be sure to notice the good things in nature too.
> *Step 3*: Upload your counts.

*Visit bigbutterflycount.
butterfly-conservation.
org to find out more.*

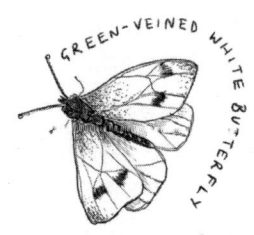

# AUGUST

August is the final month of summer, a time when greens darken or fade to a spent beige. As many fruits ripen on trees and hedgerows, autumn can feel a step away. But, while signs of the end of summer are clear, the days and evenings are often warm and humid. Wildflowers such as daisies and foxgloves should still be flowering and providing pollen for butterflies and bees. Insects of many kinds will be busy. Closer to ponds and waterways, dragonfly numbers reach their peak, bringing yet more magic to the air as they search for prey. Any swifts remaining will leave soon as autumnal migrations begin. Tired and less territorial after the breeding season, birds decrease their singing, but robins and wrens can still be heard. By the coast it's a good month to see dolphins and maybe whales and sharks too.

My nature journal notes attempt to capture this turning point in the year:

> *The August silence of the birds. Woodland paths were webbed, the leaves damp with dew. Dark shaded trunks contrasted with the bright summer light and the birds were as quiet and hidden as mammals. A*

*sparrowhawk, straight tail trailing, drifted by, and then a blackbird, as silent as the clouds across the blue. It all spiralled my thoughts, as vaporous clouds formed lines and butterflies crossed like birch leaves released. A burst dandelion seed rode unseen air, and higher, another, with its own direction.*

## Night and day

After the long evenings of summer, August reminds us that it cannot last. The tilt of the Earth on its axis and its journey about the sun inevitably shorten the day. As non-human life reacts, so do we. It has long been known that light levels can affect our mood and mental health. The reasons for this are interesting: firstly, exposing our bodies to sunlight increases the release of the mood-boosting hormone serotonin; but our preference for sunshine could also have deeper origins, perhaps a legacy from our evolution when sunnier days were safer, the light enabling predators and dangers to be seen more easily, and the heat of the sun keeping us pleasantly warm. Even today, people tend to associate light with positive emotions and darkness with negativity.

Just as we evolved to make sense of the natural world, we evolved deeply in tune with the rhythms of the day. The cycles of the day and night are ingrained within our bodies: the biological clock in our brains is connected to our retinas, so daylight is a cue that calibrates our circadian rhythm, regulating sleep and wakefulness.

Another way sunshine interacts with our bodies is through the production of vitamin D. Indeed, sunlight is our major natural source of this crucial vitamin. Vitamin D helps the body absorb essential nutrients and protects against a number of diseases; it is also thought to be beneficial for mental health.

Fundamentally, humans are diurnal; we are active in the daytime, sleepy at night. We are tuned into the rise and fall of the sun, the turning of the Earth – and the phases of the moon. There's even a suggestion that the lunar cycle affects humans, being associated with changes in sleep patterns, mood, the cardiovascular and nervous systems.

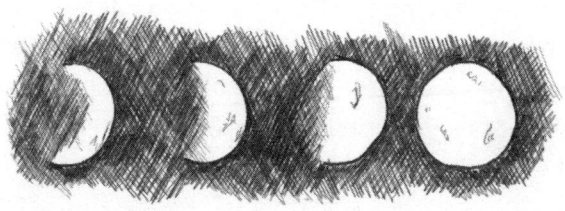

*Activity*: **Go on a dusk walk**

The warmth and earlier evenings of August present an ideal time to go on a dusk walk and experience the natural world in a magical light. Perhaps take a regular route to see how it differs at this later time, or go somewhere a little further afield: a woodland route for a mystical experience or a place with open views of the landscape and sky. As ever, whatever is comfortable and safe for you. Make sure you're visible, equipped with a torch, and an extra layer of clothing, and ensure your location doesn't have gates that might be locked at dusk!

1. Depending on how far you plan to go, start your walk 30 minutes or an hour or so before sunset on a sunny day. Then you'll be able to enjoy the 'golden hour', a time when the sun casts a warm light that transforms landscapes and highlights textures.

2. As darkness creeps across the sky, watch the colours change and be on the lookout for the bright dot of a star or planet. Perhaps you'll see birds returning to their roost or a bat flying by.

3. Many birds fall quiet in August, but listen for the changing sounds, alarm calls, perhaps an owl's hoot being carried on the cooling air.

## The long view

All of us will be aware of being part of a thread through time. From our parents, grandparents, great-grandparents on, back through 10,000 generations or so, each has successfully produced at least one child. Ninety per cent of our ancestors were hunter-gatherers, whose very survival depended upon a deep understanding of nature. They were co-dwellers on Earth, along with wildlife and trees, as part of a dynamic whole, and there was likely no concept of a separate 'nature'. If they did have any concept of nature, they would perhaps have seen it in a parental role, the giver of food and shelter like a trusted mother or father; a cooperative rather than exploitative relationship, in which nature's gifts were recognised and repaid.

It is thought that hunter-gatherers managed to meet their nutritional needs through a few hours of unhurried activity each day. But as populations grew and farming slowly spread – and with the weather and 'pests' potentially threatening a good harvest – nature became something to control and manage. Food was no longer received from a giving 'parent', but the result of hard work. Rather than having a cooperative relationship with their co-dwellers in the natural world, humans transferred their affiliation to gods who, if satisfied, might deliver a bountiful harvest.

Fast forward many generations to fourth-century Britain, where existence was hard; but even so, remarkably, people survived and procreated, giving each of us an unbroken thread back through time. The people of those times were far less embedded in the natural world than their hunter-gatherer forebears, but they still had a strong relationship with it. They saw nature as alive and enchanted; they were outside often, and surrounded by much more wildlife than we see today.

And then another revolution came along and shifted beliefs to a more recognisable modern mindset. Seventeenth-century Europe saw the dawn of the Age of Enlightenment, when concepts of individualism and self-awareness took hold, and with these a separation of the mental and the physical, and human and nature. An important catalyst in the development of this dualistic thinking was Descartes' mind-body theory. You'll recognise his famous statement, 'I think therefore I am', which signalled a dramatic shift in consciousness to reason and self-reliance. The mind became supreme – rather than our bodies being in a relationship with the world, we started to relate to the world through knowledge, from information delivered to our heads by bodily organs.

The Age of Enlightenment in turn provided the foundation for the scientific and industrial revolutions that spread throughout Europe and beyond, reinforcing the dualistic mindset. The advance of industrialisation facilitated ever greater control and exploitation of the natural world. The first factories appeared and people moved to the ever-growing towns for work, breaking the bonds with nature further still. And so it continued to the present day, when we are not just disconnected from nature but becoming ever more socially isolated, despite being surrounded by others. We've gone from nomadic social hunter-gatherer groups to digital nomads working remotely.

Humans are social animals; this is as true now as it was in hunter-gatherer times. Connections and belonging enable us to survive and thrive. Indeed, isolation and loneliness are bad for our health. Connections with nature provide a sense of belonging and a buffer against the effects of social isolation. Research has shown that people living in areas with more trees and green space tend to have a greater sense of community. Having more opportunities to get into high-quality natural settings encourages us to get out of our homes and forge relationships with neighbours.

## *Activity*: A social forage for blackberries

This activity echoes our hunter-gatherer heritage. Foraging for blackberries is a simple way to slow down, feel closer to your food and connect with both nature and the distant past.

### *Embrace the social aspect*
- Research a location. Good blackberrying spots were once a valued part of local knowledge, but the activity is less popular now. Hopefully you can find someone willing to share their knowledge with you. Or take a wander around some likely locations you've explored during the year.
- Gather a small tribe. Invite a couple of friends or family members.
- Share the bounty. Leave plenty for wildlife. Pick enough for a couple of pies or crumbles; eat one together, give the other away.

*Connect*

- Immerse your senses. As you forage, engage with the sights, sounds and scents around you. Picking fruit is a great way to slip into a mindful moment, especially when you are focused on avoiding the thorns!
- Recognise and acknowledge the wonder of the web of life you're participating in. Berries are a gift of nature that can nourish both you and the wider natural world.
- Imagine generations of your ancestors foraging for food and the pleasure they likely found tasting the fruits of summer.

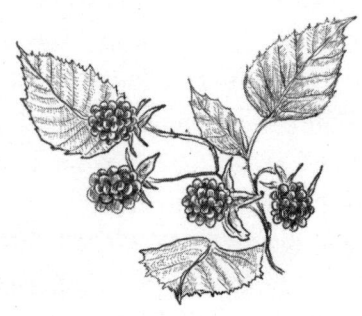

*Remember*

Before picking and eating, be 100% sure they are blackberries. They should be a familiar fruit, but if in doubt, don't. Also, only forage in publicly accessible areas. Respect private property and avoid fruit in areas where pesticides might have been sprayed, such as arable fields. Or those growing near a busy road or close to the ground, where a dog might have raised its leg. It's a good idea to visit after a bout of rain and to wash your harvest.

## Creativity

Nature is inspirational, fuelling creativity and imagination in many ways. Research has shown that higher levels of nature connection bring more innovative and divergent thinking and original creative performance.

Although important in areas like science, engineering and medicine, creativity is a word perhaps most often associated with art – all forms of art, from music, poetry and sculpture to literature and architecture. Our next activity is focused on art in its simplest form – drawing, making marks and lines. Like writing, drawing has health benefits. It affects what we see, and aids memory and recall. Sketching requires attention, which slows things down and helps manage our moods. However, while expressive – as opposed to observational or factual – writing brings the most benefits, the evidence suggests that the reverse is true for drawing. Observational drawing is about looking more closely rather than expressing feelings.

### *Activity*: Draw

Grab a pencil and a pad and head some place to sketch. Settle down close to a joy of nature, large or small. Start simply, observe, draw the shapes, lines and light. Use the drawing activity as a way to help you look closely, to notice differences. And remember, just draw what you see. Your drawing doesn't need to be accurate or good; it's the process and noticing that matter. Your image can be simple, complex, shaded or plain. Develop your own style. Once you've had a bit of practice, you can also add drawings to your nature journal.

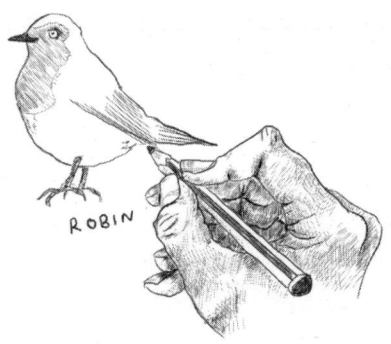

ROBIN

## Angel: The robin

Is there anything left to be said about our beloved robin, the UK's favourite bird with its familiar red breast? Robins sing most of the year to defend their territory, and by August their delightful tune rings out like a lament for the end of summer. Robins often join us in the garden or on walks, perhaps following us through a hedgerow. This isn't out of friendliness – they follow people just as they used to follow the wild boar that once roamed the land, flushing food into view as they grubbed the ground. As well as being strongly associated with Christmas, robins are common in folk-lore, a symbol of happiness and joy, a messenger from loved ones.

## *For nature*: Take part in a beach clean or litter pick

Litter is more than a mess; it can be a danger to wild-life through entanglement and chemical contamina-tion. So volunteering to pick it up is very worthwhile. Some beach cleans are more than a simple tidy-up; they take place regularly and provide useful citizen science data. Several organisations offer advice or run them, for example Surfers Against Sewage, Keep Britain Tidy and the National Trust. Remember that volunteering brings its own benefits, not least because it involves socialising. Search online and join a group near you.

# September

September is the first month of autumn. An abundance of fruit and berries hangs from trees and hedgerows. The migration of birds is at its peak, as swallows and warblers head south and skeins of geese cross the skies. If the weather is fair, this month can still feel like summer, with warm and dry days amplified by the soft, golden sun. But, as you wander woodlands, you will notice the leaves starting to transition from green to the classic colours of autumn; and perhaps, in the distance, you might start to hear the deep calls of rutting deer. As dusk falls, if you're still and silent, you might spot badgers hunting for nuts, berries and earthworms about their sett. Later still, the longer nights may bring clearer skies, enabling a better view of the stars.

These notes of mine attempt to capture that September feeling:

> *September was warm and reflective. The river flowed like light itself, individual brightnesses further diffused by the leaves of a hanging willow. A fish leapt and fell with the sound of a pearl dropped into water.*

*Thistledown spread across the plain, untroubled by the teasing air, patient and content as the lazy flight of the heron. A few days later at Brankley, the ash and larch trees took on a September shine which hid the decay below. Spires of browned foxgloves stood vertical in the light of the forest floor. Shafts of sunlight printed the leaf litter like water lilies on a pool. Leaving the wood, trees to the fore were clear and dimensioned, those afar hazed by a blue vapour of constant September sun. It was a landscape in calm, with occasional breaks of birdsong preventing a fall into dream.*

## Landscape preference

Nature exists within a landscape. So far during our year, we've tended to consider individual natural elements, such as birds and trees, dotted about a wider landscape. For many of us in the UK, whether we're urban or rural, our closest 'natural' landscape will be farmland. There may be pockets of woodland and, in some areas, moorland; and around the edge of the British Isles is a coastal landscape, of course. But there is little wilderness. Next time you're crossing the landscape on a train, look out of the window for any land that isn't managed in some way.

Just as we evolved to make sense of the natural world,

we evolved and became adapted to particular landscapes. It is thought that the preference for open views relates back to our ideal environment being the savanna-like landscape inhabited by early humans in Africa, with its resource-rich open spaces and occasional trees providing a combination of open views and refuge – offering the chance to look for food, spot predators and hide! Some researchers, however, have found modern humans prefer a rainforest over savannah, which might be explained by the rich vegetation, or by the alternative evolutionary view that early humans evolved or foraged in forests rather than open spaces.

Either way, the evolutionary influence has long since been overwritten by the here and now, our modern habitats replaced by the landscapes that people are most familiar with, or conditioned to – the rolling countryside of a green and pleasant land, for example. We all have our own likes and dislikes, and our preference for landscapes is influenced by emotional and aesthetic factors: beauty, wilderness, scale, naturalness, complexity, tranquillity, safety, mystery and awesomeness. Reducing landscapes to factors and elements in order to understand them is interesting, but something gets lost; the simplicity of our need for natural spaces, their colours, shapes and textures, feel good. The vastness and beauty trigger inspiration, wonder and meaningful memories.

How we perceive a landscape is also influenced by our level of nature connection; those with a deeper connection tending to favour forests for their potential for mystery and restoration, for example. Interestingly, the residents of countries with more arable land tend to have higher levels of nature connection than those living in countries with more pastureland. Smaller community farming is linked to a closer relationship with nature because individuals are exposed to more wildlife and become more involved with natural processes, such as planting, harvesting, and caring for the land'

## *Activity*: Visit a viewpoint

This activity involves spending some time at a place overlooking a landscape. A mountain may come to mind, but a modest hilltop or just some higher ground will do. Whatever you choose, be mindful of your safety and choose a viewpoint that is accessible and suitable for you. A place with some sense of openness, where you can linger and ponder the scale of the natural world. To begin with, try to embrace the entire panorama without focusing on anything in particular. Let the expansive view highlight the limitlessness of your mind and reveal the depth of your connection to nature.

Then, try and read the landscape. Enjoy the space, colours and contours. Trace the rivers and tracks, our own rivers of human habit across the landscape. Consider the woodlands, communities and dwellings. How is the land used: are there mainly fields of crops or areas of livestock grazing? How urban is the landscape? Are there many homes for wildlife and places for people to connect with nature? Watch the clouds and how the changing light describes the landscape. Ask yourself which elements strike you as beautiful or awe-inspiring. What thoughts and feelings does being there bring?

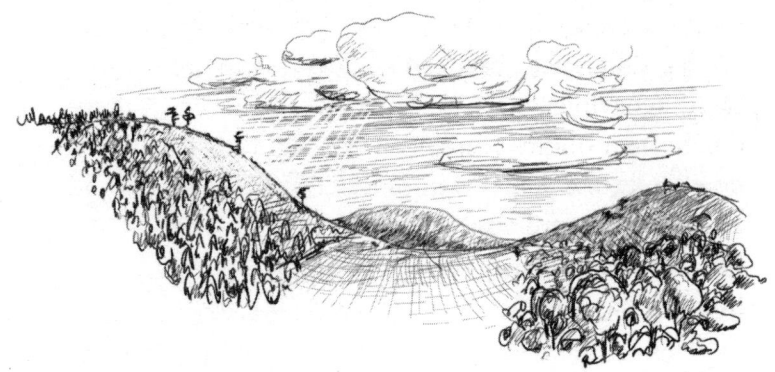

## Kinship with plants

Animals get far more attention than plants. Our visual attention is biased towards animals and we are better able to name them than plants – hence the term 'plant blindness', used to describe the tendency of people not to notice the plants in their environment. People who fail to see plants tend to just group them together into a green backdrop. Indeed, some people do not even perceive plants as living things. Trees, however, are more valued and appreciated, and seem to have a far greater everyday presence in people's lives and a deeper cultural significance. And we may enjoy flowers. It's the wider plant world that tends to go unseen.

Why is it that a kinship with mammals is easier than

a kinship with a dandelion? In the tree of life, plants and animals separated a billion years or more ago. However, there is commonality. Both animals and plants need nutrients, water, light and heat to sustain energy and life. Animals are obviously mobile in that search, but plants too steer themselves towards the light. And, while there are big differences between the two, there are comparable behaviours and features. As we saw in August, our human bodies respond to the light, just as plants do, thanks to distant evolutionary features retained and adapted over millennia. The science is complex, but there's a serious suggestion that the gut–brain axis in humans has an evolutionary link to the root–leaf axis in plants.[27]

## *Activity*: Watch roots grow

Keeping a 'pet plant' and monitoring its progress daily has been found to increase our appreciation of plants and our connection with them. This activity is a little different from the earlier growing activity as it involves taking herb cuttings and watching their roots grow – the root–leaf axis. The cuttings can be taken from potted herbs from the supermarket or from a plant you're already growing.

You'll need:

- fresh herbs – basil, mint, oregano or parsley tend

to work
- scissors
- a clean glass jar
- water.

Instructions:

1. Select a stem with several sets of healthy leaves.
2. Use clean scissors to cut off 10–15cm sprigs just below a leaf node (where a leaf meets the stem). Remove the lower leaves, leaving two or three at the top.
3. Add clean water to the jar, leaving a few centimetres of space at the top.
4. Place the stem ends of your cuttings into the water, taking care not to submerge any leaves.
5. Place the jar on a windowsill that gets plenty of sunshine.
6. Wait a few days. Soon, you should see tiny white roots emerging from the stems. Changing the water every two or three days can help to prevent rot.
7. Monitor their progress, watching how the roots emerge and grow.
8. Once the roots are about 3–5cm long, your cuttings are ready for transplanting.
9. Fill small pots with well-draining potting

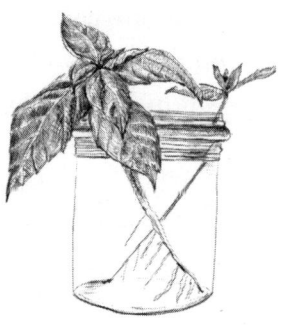

compost. Carefully plant the cuttings in the pots, keeping the roots intact. Water well and return to their sunny spot.

10. Once your herbs are established in the pots, you can start snipping leaves to use.

## Beyond being human

Through the past months, we've considered noticing nature, its impact on our emotions and the various ways in which we humans connect with it. We've also progressed into deeper aspects around the meaning of nature. Let us return, for a moment, to the idea of our shared place in nature and beliefs – a place which ultimately depends on transcending a human-centred view of the world.

Anthropomorphism is the practice of attaching human characteristics to non-human things, both animate and inanimate. This is an everyday occurrence across cultures and histories. From religion to video games via vacuum cleaners, there are countless examples of wildlife and objects being given a human-type character or essence.

Anthropomorphism has its good sides. It can help us appreciate the wonders of the non-human world. Indeed, it tends to be practised more by people who have a closer relationship with nature, and it can help strengthen pro-nature behaviour through increasing empathy.

The problem is that as humans, we are biased, and in looking at the world through our human-centred glasses, we project our worldview onto everything we see and assume that animals think and feel like us, which has the potential to distort reality.

This desire to bestow things with a human essence has parallels with the Western understanding of animism. Animists believe that all entities have a unique spiritual essence. This essence animates living beings and natural elements such that no stone is just a stone, no flower just a flower; everything has unique individuality and spirit. From this perspective, each tree, even each leaf, can affect us in different ways.

However, animism is very different from anthropomorphism, which only sees things in terms of being human – humanness bringing value. Animism sees no distinction between the physical and spiritual world; rather, there is a universal natural energy or spirit that runs through everything. The animistic worldview likely has roots in hunter-gatherer beliefs, which would have been challenged as humans increasingly turned to farming and animals became objects with a purpose. So much so that its notions of animating essences and stones with unique spirits may now seem fanciful and far from science. Yet, quantum mechanics tells us that at the subatomic level there is a whole realm of connections between particles, such as fermions, bosons, quarks and leptons. The more science discovers, the more mysteries it seems to open up. Take, for example, 'dark matter', undiscovered matter which doesn't interact with ordinary matter.

There's potentially a lot going on within a stone.

When you think about scientists searching for hidden particles, the idea of a universal natural energy seems less fanciful. Also, at the microscopic scale, there are many interactions between the human body and the rest of the natural world that challenge the prevailing view. For example, most of our health institutions in the Western world see people as separate from their environment: we are bodies, or minds, to be treated and repaired when we fall ill. And yet our bodies are complex systems, involving a whole range of mechanical, chemical and electrochemical interactions. Our breath exhales chemicals and our bodies produce electro-magnetic fields that can be detected outside the body. Likewise, our bodies receive signals via specialised cells that make up our senses. Chemical and electrical signals change physical reality into the content of our brains: a single drop of cool rain on our face becomes a sensation, a ripple on the film of consciousness. Also rippling the pool are sights and sounds. Photons from the sun are transformed into visions in our minds, and changes in the air vibrate through ossicle and incus to provide a soundtrack to that vision.

In Western minds, animism is often grossly misunderstood and seen as a primitive belief system under which things such as trees and stones are conscious in some way. These sorts of ideas are inevitably going to seem odd to a human-centred society for which agency is about minds, personality and mental capacity. Arguably, animism conceptualises agency with far more subtlety and intelligence; for animists, agency is about relationships between things, not a quality found within things. It is more about communication and interaction based on a systematic understanding of how animals, plants and other non-human things perceive, respond and communicate. So, agency is exhibited by a wide range of natural things appropriate to their existence. Animism is natural. Think of how children demonstrate animistic thinking, only to be taught this is as an 'error' in our rationalistic world. The perceived agency of a child's much-loved teddy bear comes from the relationship they have formed with it. Perhaps the same can be said for your favourite tree?

Animism rejects the human reference point, taking an eco-centred perspective instead. And it can offer a compelling and important view of the natural world at a time when new ways of relating to ecosystems are needed. Rather than challenge modern scientific knowledge, animism anticipates or converges with recent trends in Western science, such as the biology of consciousness, extended mind and embodied cognition, where the wider environment and our minds operate in union.

## *Activity*: A kind of animism

Hopefully, after nine months cultivating awareness and connecting with the rest of nature, you are more than ready to accept the interconnectedness of all things and perhaps their invisible essence, which incidentally can be whatever you want it to be – bosons, quarks or spirit. During your daily interactions with nature, be conscious of that hidden essence.

Embracing an animistic outlook changes the way we interact with the world. Just as we're polite and considerate to other humans, we can be considerate to the non-human world, acknowledging the flower we're about to pick or the fruit we harvest. When planting a tree or flower, rather than impose your own will, decide and agree its position based on your relationship with the land as part of a respectful interaction.

Your newfound connections have likely already led to a greater respect for all beings. You doubtless have a greater sense of gratitude for the world around you. Everything is special in its own way, something you've perhaps felt before when placing a pebble or shell in your pocket and taking it home with you, feeling it within your palm as you go. Develop rituals that honour nature and are meaningful to you and make them part of your daily or seasonal routine. There is no right or wrong; animism can be a deeply personal practice.

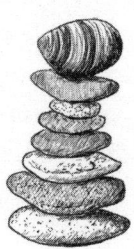

## Angel: The house sparrow

Where there are people there are often sparrows. They are the most widespread bird in the world; however, their numbers have declined sharply in the UK, so it is important to conserve their preferred habitat and provide nesting sites. Sparrows are resourceful opportunists, eating a varied diet of grains, scraps and insects, thus helping to protect both crops and gardens. They are social birds that live in tight-knit communities that can be woven into the fabric of our lives. Their distinctive chatter is often heard from within a dense hedge or shrub. Enjoy their social interactions and regular dust bathing. The presence of sparrows brings a touch of joy to our days.

## *For nature*: A log pile ecosystem

A simple pile of logs left undisturbed can provide essential food and shelter for all sorts of creatures, creating a miniature ecosystem and supporting wider biodiversity in your garden or local community. It will also help control some of the insects that might be eating your vegetables. Community gardens, parks and nature reserves often welcome volunteers to help create and maintain areas for wildlife. Check with your local noticeboards or contact local nature organisations to find opportunities near you.

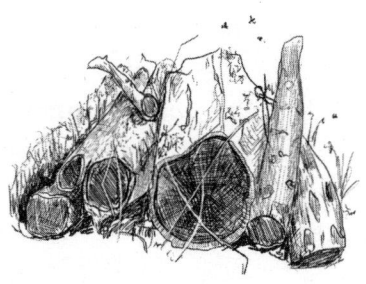

Here are some tips for making a log pile:

1. Gather materials. Look for a variety of recently fallen branches and twigs. If you are away from home, get permission and don't remove wood that's been there a while – it's likely a home already.
2. Find a shady corner. A spot near a wall or under a bush is ideal. You can dig a small hole if you wish so that your log pile emerges from the ground, creating a wider variety of habitats.
3. Build your haven. Stack the branches to form a sturdy structure. If you've dug out some soil, it can always be placed on top.
4. Wait. Much like a bug hotel, your creation will gradually come alive as insects, spiders and beetles move in. Log piles are a little different, though, as they can be left to become damp and rot, attracting amphibians like toads and newts. The larger gaps might be favoured by mice,

hedgehogs or even a wren. A damp area around a log pile can be good for fungi too.

5. Integrate. If you'd like the log pile to feel more of a part of the garden, you can surround it with a few native wildflowers that enjoy a shady spot, or some spring-flowering bulbs. Or cover it with a honeysuckle.

# OCTOBER

The colours of autumn reach their glorious peak in October, the golden hues of the day contrasting with the ever-longer nights. During those nights, you are more likely to hear the twit-twoo of tawny owls, which are at their most vocal as they establish and defend their territory. Fieldfare and redwing return from areas such as Scandinavia and Eastern Europe in search of berries to eat. Swans and geese flock to wetlands. One of the few plants to start to flower is ivy; when the sun shines, a decent patch of ivy will be busy with insects collecting the last nectar and pollen of the year. Below them, hedgehogs will be preparing to hibernate, eating more and finding a safe spot to spend the winter. Within the fallen leaves, mushrooms and fungi will appear.

An October entry from my nature diary explores the wonder of autumnal trees in my local patch of woodland:

> *At Brook Hollows, the wind released leaves into the lake from high on the sycamore. Some spiralled down, stalk first to puncture the water and then float, bobbing and*

*pecking at the water like the fowl beyond. The willow launched canoe-like forms that stayed afloat, crossing the lake on the breeze to gather in the bay of the isle. Meanwhile, above, gulls gathered in an apery of discontent. The normally dark stream threaded through drifts of lime, becoming a flow of highlighted bronze that wrapped itself in gold. On land, the clearings were more leaf than earth and a decoration of fallen ash challenged the gloom. A beech harboured light within its distributed branches, its calmness of space lighting the fading leaves to a revival. The thin dark branches spanned an area of woodland out of proportion to their slender girth. It is a tree that could shelter a choir, but neither they, nor a blackbird, could sing its compelling form.*

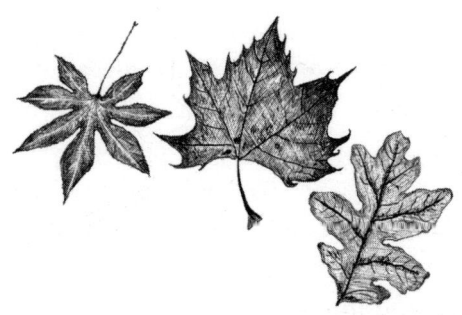

## Invisible friends

We've seen how nature looks after us, flowing through our senses and calming our bodies to bring wellbeing. But as we saw in the last chapter, to really connect with nature, we need to get to a beyond-human understanding of the way we relate to the world around us. Everything is related and we are just a node within an entangled web of relationships too complex to ever fully understand.

Our focus through the months so far has been sensory contact with nature. We've seen how the body responds when we simply look at flowers. Sound, such as birdsong, is another rich sensory pathway, and we've seen how hearing nature can reduce stress. Similarly, touching nature, for example, wood, calms the body. We've looked at the benefits to our wellbeing of natural foods and natural odours, such as the scents of flowers. These are all sensory experiences that we are conscious of and can enjoy. Let's now explore some of our non-sensory relationships, such as the one we have with microbes.

Microbes are our invisible friends. We can't see, taste, hear or touch them, but they are everywhere, inside us and out. Each one of us consists of half-human and half-microbial cells. It's a relationship that plays a vital role in our health and very being. Our gut microbiome, for example, is linked to our brain, influencing our thinking and moods.

Humans are, quite literally, a walking symbiotic

community that depends upon continual interactions within and beyond the skin. Trillions of microorganisms, such as bacteria, fungi and viruses, live on and within us, and the vast majority of them are good for us. So it seems very strange that we are encouraged to banish bacteria from our homes and bodies. Unprocessed whole foods often contain good bacteria, as does the soil they grew in. Even growing lettuce indoors has been found to provide a meaningful boost in bacterial diversity, which is important for the development and function of the immune system. Contact with microbe-rich soil is beneficial for health.[28] Trees also play an important role in the species richness of bacteria as demonstrated by the interesting fact that despite hosting more species of bacteria, a woodland contains fewer pathogens than an urban sports field.

Nature connects with us in many ways, seen and unseen. And incidentally, it's not all about microbes. There are plenty of other invisible, non-sensory pathways to nature connection. With each breath, we inhale thousands of organisms. Back in May, we explored some of the benefits of forest bathing, including breathing in phytoncides, the natural organic compounds given off by trees, which are actually believed to be *anti*microbial and enhance immune system activity. Another non-sensory route is negative air ions. These are produced when an electron is released by one gas molecule and captured by another. The energy needed for this process can come from cosmic rays, thunder and waterfalls, so they are more abundant in natural places. It is thought that these ions could be linked to wellbeing and mood. A simple breath is a route to a closer relationship with our invisible friends.

## *Activity*: Breathe

This simple activity is as fundamental and universal as they come. Taking a breath is an essential first moment. Air is the breath of the flesh of the Earth. It carries our first words and the stories we tell. Inhaled, it nourishes our own flesh.

Visit the most ancient woodland you can easily reach. A place where each step compresses the leaves of a thousand summers. Microbes fill the air and each breath. Wander until the trees suggest a place to stand. For a few minutes, breathe in through your nose, counting to four slowly. Feel the air enter and your chest rise and hold your breath for another count of four. Slowly breathe out through your mouth for a count of four. With each breath, imagine you're drawing in an array of tiny friends that thrive in this woodland. Feel the air fill your lungs, carrying them deep within your body, some joining your own internal ecosystem.

Whether you stand or wander through the woodland, bring your attention to its sounds. Sounds carried by the air, invisible waves emanating from their source. Focus on the scent of the woodland, more unseen molecules carried on the air. Feel the touch of the breeze on your skin, breathe in the out-breath of the trees, share the air with the animals and birds. From the atomic essence of matter within the trees to the microscopic matter within a simple breath, wonder at the world. Capture your thoughts and feelings for your journal. Write about the images that come to mind.

## Drama and song

Art – whether it be drawing, painting, music, story-telling, drama, songwriting, poetry, dance, photography, filmmaking or sculpture – offers multiple opportunities for exploring your own relationship with nature. When studies were conducted with children and young people engaging in these activities, all of them experienced a positive impact, feeling that nature was becoming part of their identity. The process of change is thought to come in many ways. Clearly, creating art requires noticing and engagement with nature, which we've already seen is essential to nature connection. It requires imagination and creativity to develop the concept. And it requires working outside, being free from the indoor norms.

We've looked at drawing and photography as approaches to nature connection. This time, you might want to branch out. You could gather some friends to make music in the woods. Outdoor music-making has been found in studies to create a heightened state of awareness and spiritual moments as people enter a new world in harmony with nature. A very different level of connection to, say, going on a nature trail which includes maps, nature facts and checkpoints. Three make a choir – there's nothing like singing in the woods on a still autumnal evening (and breathing in all those microbes and phytoncides). You might even stage a concert. You could write a play inspired by a natural setting, or a view. Think of *A Midsummer Night's Dream* – with its enchanted forest where real and spiritual worlds collide.

## *Activity*: A nature-inspired artwork

This activity gives you free rein to be creative and slow! Give yourself as long as you want: a whole month is fine, and try to create your work outside in nature as much as possible. It can be helpful, when thinking of an artistic approach to nature connection, to be aware of the 'head, heart and hand framework' – the head providing discovery through understanding, learning and critical reflection; the heart being about attunement through emotions and relational knowing; and the hands about flow, the psychomotor domain of skill, deep engagement and 'in the moment' actions.[29]

### *Gather inspiration*
The first two steps involve your head and heart. Seek out and discover something new about nature or your relationship with it, something that you find emotional or meaningful. This can be a sensory exploration close to home or gathering inspiration from another landscape or from a variety of sources, such as a natural

history museum. You could look back at previous months for inspiration or explore a particular aspect of nature connection. This process can include gathering natural materials where it is OK and safe to do so. If you struggle for inspiration, a simple approach is to create a collage, something beautiful from items you find, such as feathers, fallen leaves and seed heads.

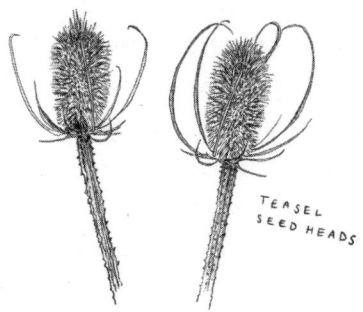

TEASEL SEED HEADS

## Concept

After discovery and understanding comes the concept for your artwork. Whether you're exploring your own relationship with nature or expressing what you've discovered or an environmental concern, you now need to settle on your medium, be that painting, music, film or sculpture. Your concept could grow into a community-based project involving many hands to bring wider connection with nature or communicate a local, nature-related issue.

## Create

Now you can explore and develop your concept and skills, perhaps actively through testing out some ideas. Give yourself plenty of time to engage with your work and immerse yourself in it – ideally outdoors.

## *Activity*: Get to know a tree

Month by month through the year, you have been focusing on one particular tree, from winter sleep, through spring awakening and the leaves harbouring summer sunshine. The fresh leaves of spring will have darkened over the summer before taking on their autumnal hue as the tree prepares for winter. Track the changing leaf colours, how they vary. And how frequently the leaves fall. Gather a few fallen leaves: what do they tell you of summer and the spent energy of spring?

## Angel: The rook

Rooks are wonderful birds. They are highly social, and outside of the early-spring breeding season, they gather in large flocks to feed on worms, seeds and insects. In October, these flocks can be found in dormant fields, like notes on staves of cut rows playing autumn. As evening approaches, they often rise and circle before returning to their rookeries to roost communally.

These regular daily movements are worth looking out for. There are interesting accounts of people's relationships with rooks. For example, Esther Woolfson found a common world with them, realising what we share, from backbone and brain structures to senses and social behaviour.[30] To some, unaware of the birds' propensity for affection and amusement, their harsh voices might represent dark forces. We humans often make judgements based on perceived 'otherness' and superstition. But when I hear the rook bleed its call into the air of the changing season, my heart heals. Watch as they swirl about the rookery trees with what seems like glee, their blackness morphing and constantly shifting shape.

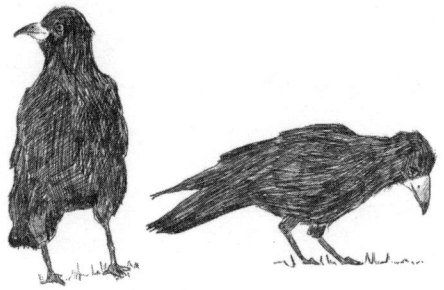

### *For nature*: **Be messy**

If you have a garden there's always an urge to tidy up – to clear away the remnants of summer and fallen leaves of autumn. Similarly, you may see your local park or community space being tidied. Yet the 'mess' can be a haven for wildlife. As well as doing things in your garden, you could ask if a local patch can be left for nature. Here are some tips for nurturing some natural habitats to help insects, birds and small mammals through the winter:

- Wild edges. Allow the edges of your garden to be a little wild. Unruly plants, long grass and tangled shrubs can provide shelter.
- Leave some seed heads. Don't deadhead or cutback all flowers, especially if there are seed heads on plants such as sunflowers and teasels that provide a seasonal feast for birds.
- Leaves and twigs. Resist the urge to tidy away every leaf and twig. Gather a pile in a secluded corner, under hedges or bushes, or add them to your log pile to provide additional shelter, insulation and even a potential spot for a hedgehog to hibernate. As their usual diet declines, hedgehogs look for cosy spots in which to bed in for the winter.
- Collect pond leaves. This is in fact a tidying tip! While a mess can be good, avoid letting leaves accumulate in a pond, because they can upset the balance of the pond's mini ecosystem as they decompose.

Remember, the more we can help wildlife through the winter, the more there will be to enjoy next spring.

# NOVEMBER

Autumn gradually becomes winter in November. Long nights and colder conditions return and those changes bring different experiences. With strong winds, most trees will be bare, but on a woodland walk you can still find colour and brightness through fallen leaves, fungi, acorns and chestnuts. It can be easier to spot lichens too. Garden birdfeeders will get busier, perhaps with some new visitors, such as redpolls, bramblings or siskins, among the usual favourites. Blackbirds and song thrushes will be hopping about searching for worms and fallen berries. In the field, corvids, such as rooks and jackdaws, will gather. By the coast, large flocks of waders can be seen. Autumn is also a peak time for grey seal pups.

This is a November entry from my nature journal:

> *It was mid-November and frost emphasised the form and structure of the lying leaves. Bare birch trunks became beams of light, speared by the dark arrows of their branches. Fieldfares massed from field to tree, from tree to shrub, until they rose as one, occupying*

*the sky that spoke of winter and the setting
of the sun. A blackbird lost of voice perched
where it had once found song, receiving the
rain with a steady contentment, as if each
drop were a note for the coming year.*

## Virtual nature

As days shorten and winter takes hold, getting out and
noticing nature can be more of a challenge. Fortunately,
and especially for those with limited mobility, virtual
tools can provide an alternative way to engage with
nature. These can range from immersive experiences
using a headset to more modest engagement through
watching a video. Virtual can also be film of real or
simulated nature, the benefit of the latter being that
nature doesn't have to be disturbed by human presence
to make it.

It's early days for research into the impact of immersive virtual reality on nature connection, but there
are positive signs that it can improve it, albeit less so
than contact with real nature. As for watching videos
of nature, there is evidence that this too can lead to a
short-term boost in nature connection, although not as
much as an immersive experience.

It does appear that we can be tricked by simulated
nature. But there is also need for care. Might simula-
tion raise expectations such that real nature disap-
points and thereby loses its value? Could our search for

simplicity and perfection lead to surrounding ourselves with simulated nature, as already seen with the growing popularity of plastic plants and lawns?

### *Activity*: Nature's gallery

With the arrival of darker evenings, this activity invites you to connect with nature through a personal lens – your photographs of nature. Gather a collection of your nature photos through the year, ones you're particularly pleased with or that remind you of a special moment with nature. With digital cameras and smartphones it has never been easier to view, select and sort photographs – although the sheer number can be a problem! There are also many services available to help you turn your photos into books, calendars or simple prints.

- *Gather and sort.* Revisit your pictures from the year, allowing yourself to be transported back to the moment, place and feeling they captured. Reflect on what drew you to record the moment, what you noticed, or a story related to the image.
- *Create groups.* You can sort your photos and create albums simply by month or season; you could also arrange them by landscape theme (woodland, views, coastal scenes) or according to their emotional content (separating images that induce calm from those that evoke excitement or a darker mood, for example), or

meaning, (those with a story to tell).

- *Reflection*. Take some time to reflect on your collection. Which photos mean the most to you? Which bring you the most joy or calm?
- *Share*. Perhaps share your favourite photo and its story with a friend or create a physical or a digital album for the year.
- *Look ahead*. Select an aspect of nature you'd like to focus on next year.

## Storytelling

Billions of photos are taken each year, the vast majority stored on phones or computers, servers and the like. That data stores our stories. How long will it survive? Will it be accessible to our descendants?

Stories, folklore and myths can be evocative and enduring. They are a fundamental tool for creating, sharing, and maintaining culture and also one of the key ways in which we present ourselves to others. Stories promote communication and learning, drawing people in, firing imagination and building relationships. They help organise our experiences and make sense of our lives. They are core cognitive structures linked to understanding, organisation of knowledge and memory across cultures. Having been a part of human existence for tens of thousands of years, stories are hard-wired into our brains.

Storytelling and folklore are an important part of our

relationship with nature – both good and bad. Stories create a reality that can be positive or negative. Wolves, for example, are generally portrayed as threatening and sinister. Such stereotypes matter as they inform beliefs and can create fear. These fairy tales and fear-inducing myths about the 'Big Bad Wolf' have survived through many generations and are still told by parents and teachers to children, contributing to their perceptions and worldview.

### *Activity*: Create a nature connection story

In many non-Western cultures, storytelling and folklore transmit valuable lessons about nature conservation. And even in Western communities, where oral story-telling, the traditional way of communicating down the generations, is beginning to fade away, tales and folk-lore can still be an important part of our relationship with nature. Inspired by your journal and photo gallery, create a nature connection-themed story. Your story will need to include:

- characters, either human or non-human
- a focus on emotions or essence
- causally related events
- an unexpected challenge or development
- the effect of the challenge on the characters
- a resolution that affects the characters.

Your story might aim to celebrate nature and highlight the commonalities between the reader's life and those in the natural world. You might write a story to tell a child or grandchild, one they could go on to tell to their own offspring.

## Maps

Maps tell stories about our relationship with nature too. Traditional paper maps often provide a detailed and accurate representation of the natural landscape, a helicopter view of rivers, hills, roads and settlements. They're wonderful creations, but it requires skill to get the most out of them and construct a useful image in the mind. The landscape, map and mind become connected as we try to find our way. More recently we have come to use digital street maps, which do much of the work for us, while still influencing and contributing to our thinking and actions.

Like our brains, effective maps structure information. And in the process, some information is inevitably simplified, excluded or even distorted. Maps and memory are not a perfect mirror of reality. We can easily access satellite views, but we don't use them as maps because they are full of unnecessary detail and can hide what we're looking for. A good map distributes thinking so that it isn't wholly internal or external. Good maps should make mentally imagining and evaluating actions easier.

Maps can also encourage us to pause and notice nature, help us find joy and connection. Through careful design and selection of the information to include, and even exaggerate, maps can carry messages and create meaningful journeys – ones that tap into the pathways to nature connection.

When I first started renewing my relationship with the rest of nature, one of the first things I did was draw a map of my local landscape. It stripped away the detail to reveal the basic form of the landscape, the hills and valleys. I exaggerated the hills to match how they felt on the ground – steep! I used a viewpoint that looked across the hills from high above the valley below. And slowly, without my even realising it, the map changed my understanding of my local landscape, revealing a modest plateau between two rivers. Onto that I added the places and features that meant something to me. Years later, when I think of my local landscape, I think in terms of my map and the simple context it provides.

### *Activity*: Make a nature connection map

As we've seen, maps can be much more than a tool for getting from A to B. Maps can record meaning, beauty and emotions. Create a map of a place meaningful to you. Include the detail that matters to you. Feel free to exaggerate the hills and valleys. You can also map nature's movements, the daily routine of rooks or the places where certain insects gather. Consider how maps can help:

- activate the senses through highlighting places to pause, look, listen, smell or touch.
- Elicit emotions by mapping the joy and calm of the landscape.
- Highlight places of beauty in the natural world.
- Provide and help discover meaning through using natural waypoints or adding in stories, poems and art.
- Embed actions that are good for nature and do not disturb it.

You could work with people from your community to co-create a local nature connection map, one that goes beyond facts, figures and labels to explore the pathways to nature connection.

## Beyond the moment

Many nature connection exercises focus on being mindful and 'in the moment'. What is rarely considered is the idea of looking back, or forwards, over time, which is quite odd ,given how much we can learn from the way our ancestors lived in more harmonious relationships with nature. The past makes the present meaningful; at the same time, moving beyond the present can be powerful.

Nostalgia, a sentimental desire for a former time, place or relationship, is an emotion that is frequently experienced across cultures. It is often focused on cherished memories of past experiences, rituals and traditions, the events that infuse life with meaning. It is a bridge between the past and present, an emotion that can be purposely explored to render life more meaningful.

Like nature connection, nostalgia brings positive emotions and a sense of being part of something, or some time, larger than our own here and now. Knowing something about our ancestors shapes our personal identity, connects us with a place and brings continuity. It also encourages us to look forwards and think about becoming good ancestors ourselves, by leaving the natural world, and our relationship with it, in a better place.

The diagram opposite offers a 'nature connection space' that you can refer back to as you continue to seek your own ways to deepen your connection with nature. Consider the fleetingness of the present, as represented by the mayfly, whose winged adulthood can last for just a single day. Notice how this can be the basis for a deeper state of reflection, represented by the owl and its associated wisdom. Reflecting on our relationship with nature can also take us out of the moment and back into the past, our minds roving just like the wolf that used to roam the UK. Equally, it can inspire new ideas and ways of being, getting us to think about the future and the importance of looking after nature for the generations to come; this is represented by the beaver, that magnificent tree feller, river changer and wetland creator that is now being successfully reintroduced to the UK.

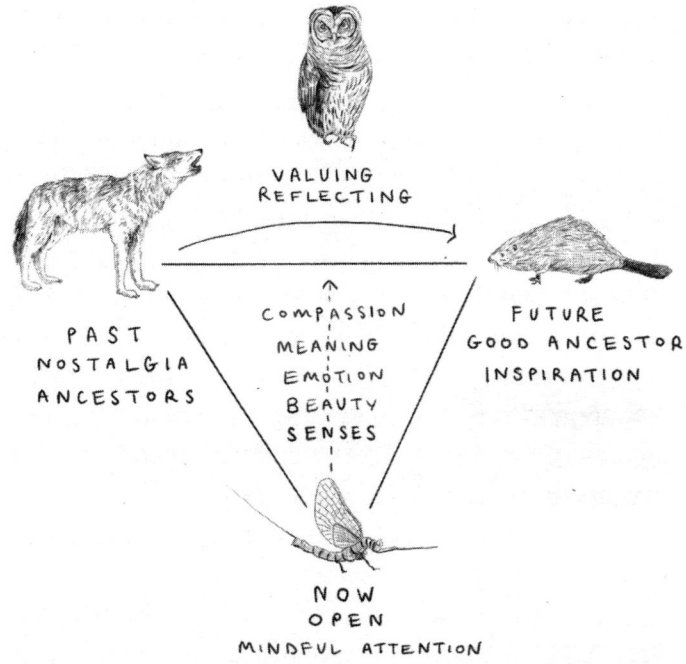

Our sense of time is interesting. Our modern lives are driven by 'mechanical time': schedules and clocks define our days. This affects how we view and value it, puts us under pressure and detaches us from natural rhythms, especially when we're in an urban environment. Research shows that people care more about the future after spending time in a natural setting than they do after spending time in an urban setting. It is also found that time feels longer when spent in nature, inducing a more balanced perspective on the flow between past, present and future. This matters, as the perceived availability of time influences our behaviours, wellbeing and future thinking.

## *Activity*: Cherishing favourite moments from the past

As an emotion tied to meaning, nostalgia is a great basis for nature connection. This activity is about looking back and bringing a past moment into the present to encourage a sense of belonging. To start, think of a favourite moment you have had with nature, a cherished memory. Consider what made that moment special, where you were, what you were doing and how you felt at the time. Imagine that scene, and perhaps find an old photograph or reconnect with someone else who was there. This can become a story in your nature journal.

## *Activity*: Time walk

As we've been creating stories and maps and considering time, let's end November by getting outside and creating a time walk, ideally in a place within easy reach, depending on your community, a footpath or ancient way, perhaps one buried beneath modernity, only revealed by an old map – many historical maps have been digitised and can be found online.

Start with a little research: how has this place changed over the last century? What was it like in Victorian times? Try to find out a fact or two for each period, back through Georgians, Stuarts and Tudors to Medieval and Saxon times. Perhaps there was a Roman road or an ancient fort nearby. With your newfound knowledge, plan a route and walk in the footsteps of our ancestors. Imagine the natural world at that time, the wolves, beavers, bears and lynx that would have been roaming. As we saw in the research earlier, the time you spend on your walk can feel longer than it actually is.

## Angel: The long-tailed tit

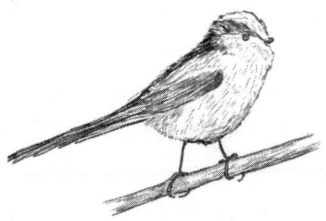

Long-tailed tits feature regularly in my nature journals. This joyful lollipop of a bird, very often spiralling branches, decorating newly bare trees and bending the uppermost twigs, is rarely alone. In gardens, parks and woodland, they will flit, float and pause in trios or more as they explore each tree and move on to the next in a constant search for food. The long-tailed tit is one of the UK's smallest birds, with a tail longer than its body. Black and white markings on the head, back and wings contrast with a pink-blushed underbelly. They are extremely social, calling to each other with a high-pitched note. They weave remarkable nests from moss, leaves and cobwebs and line them with feathers to create a cosy home for their young. You may spot one in bare hedgerows. When the cold weather arrives, long-tailed tits huddle together unseen in communal roosts.

### *For nature*: Clean your nestboxes

November, being outside the breeding season, is a good time to inspect and clean your nestboxes. Wear gloves and be sure to avoid breathing in dust and mites. You'll need a stiff brush and a mild disinfectant solution such as one part white vinegar and nine parts water.

Take down your nestbox and remove any nests. You might find unhatched eggs or dead chicks – put these in a bag inside your wheelie bin for household waste.

If it is in good repair, use your brush to remove any other debris and give it a scrub with the disinfectant solution. Then rinse it thoroughly and dry it out before rehanging. If it has not been used, you could try a new position. If it is damaged or rotting, repair it or add a new one to your Christmas list!

# DECEMBER

December brings short days, cold conditions and the start of winter. It can seem that much in nature has fallen dormant, but there's still plenty to enjoy. You might see squirrels or glimpse a fox, and birds remain our constant companions, returning to gardens and parks in greater numbers. As the light fades, look out for swirling starling murmurations. They are a real spectacle and worth seeking out. On cold nights you might find pied wagtails gathering in urban trees for extra warmth. By late December, rooks might be starting to nest. Trees will have returned to their bare form. There is also a whole layer of plant life that repays closer inspection at this time of year. Cushion mosses can bring a vibrant green to the most mundane locations, their tiny leaves just a millimetre or two long. Take a look and see if you can find small red stalks topped by a single bud-like capsule containing spores.

This December journal entry relays the end of my second nature connection year:

> *Finches peeled from the dormant hedgerows*
> *and curved with the wind to a lone oak. In*

*a nearby stream, floodwaters had thatched reeds into breaking waves. I felt I was mining words from the landscape. And within these quiet fields, I felt an end to my journey; a unity and understanding. Later, the mild air brought wonder to the longest night; a blackbird returned to song, its energy of tone defeating the buffeting breeze to enliven every space and surface; an angel bringing news of a new year.*

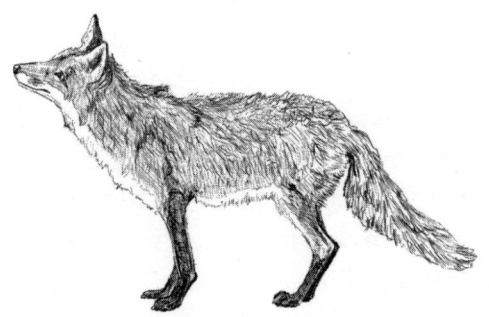

## A friend in nature

Hopefully, during the past year you have found a friend in nature. A close bond and a relationship. If we think about our relationships with people, some of them are close and others more distant. We don't evaluate these relationships by time spent together and visits made. Spending 40 hours a week with a work colleague doesn't mean we have a deeper bond with them than we do with a friend we visit one evening a month. Relationships are about love and compassion. They motivate our behaviour. We'd do more for a friend than we'd do for a stranger. We need to restore this sort of relational perspective when it comes to nature.

Thankfully, major environmental institutions have recognised this and are advocating the need to fix our failing relationship with nature. Research into human relationships show that they are built on trust, commitment, reciprocity, interdependence and intimacy. And there are many parallels between these human–human relationships and human–nature relationships. Just like relationships with friends and family, our relationship with nature can fulfil our need for belonging, shape our identity and expand our sense of self. Nature lovers are more likely to trust and make sacrifices for nature. A close relationship with nature brings similar wellbeing benefits as close relationships with people; as do acts of intimacy with nature, sensory and sensual experiences such as walking barefoot through the grass.

## *Activity*: Celebrate the winter solstice

Christmas is a time centred on relationships. We make commitments to meet friends and family. Gifts are exchanged between friends and loved ones – it's a celebration and festival of relationships in many ways.

The winter solstice, which falls a few days before Christmas on 21st December, marks the moment when the sun reaches its lowest point in the sky, bringing the shortest day and the longest night. Often called Yule, it has been celebrated for millennia across many cultures, with gatherings and feasting as people salute the returning light that follows the shortest day.

The winter solstice is a time of hope and renewal. An opportunity to connect with natural cycles. As dawn follows the longest darkness, it is a time to cast aside burdens and start anew.

Whether you follow ancient traditions or create your own, this December set out to celebrate the winter solstice. Then, as the new year approaches, plan a calendar of rituals and events. Consider holidays and trips to places with more nature to notice.

## The power of visualisation

As winter sets in, the joy of summer can seem a long way away. However, we can travel through time in our minds to a summer day at a favourite spot. One way of doing this is to listen to a narrated audio journey to help create vivid mental images of nature. These imagined experiences activate many areas of the brain in the same way that real visual experiences do: just ten minutes is enough. An imagined walk through a woodland can be quite real – and can reduce stress and anxiety, just as being in nature itself does.

## *Activity*: Time travel

Take a moment to travel in time by allowing your mind to 'go on a walk'. Picture a visit to one of your favourite places in nature at the most vibrant time of year.

- Find a place you can be comfortable and undisturbed for ten minutes. Close your eyes, relax and take a few deep breaths to calm the mind.
- Visualise the space and focus on the sensations of being in it. Take some time to look around your imagined space. Visualise the ground before you, the plants and trees. Let birds pass by and imagine their song.
- Take your place within this landscape, let your senses settle.
- Focus your attention in a particular direction, or on something with presence in your chosen landscape. A tree, perhaps, deeply rooted in the earth.
- Bring your attention to the sounds, be they birdsong, the buzz of insects, a nearby stream or simply the rustle of a gentle breeze in the trees.
- Allow yourself to relax and your senses to open. These gifts of nature are also relaxed, comfortable with themselves, accepting.
- Be absorbed by the richness of your imagined landscape. Notice the emotions evoked.
- Maintain your attention to nature. Merge your awareness of the sights and sounds, the touch of the breeze.

- Allow your mind to expand across the landscape. Become part of the landscape, notice how, as you breathe in, the land gently rises, then falls as you breathe out. Let yourself become deeply rooted in the earth and imagine your close relationship with the wildlife that surrounds you.
- Let nature's beauty wash over you, feel the wonder, the calm and joy.
- Let go of any thoughts and worries. There are no aims. There is no need to achieve.
- If your attention wanders, let it return to your imagined landscape, to engagement with the natural world.
- As you become more attuned, notice the impact of this natural landscape on your body, heart and mind. The sense of aliveness it brings. Allow yourself to be connected.
- To aid your imagining, you can play birdsong or listen to an audio guide at bit.ly/natureGI.

## Keep on noticing

Although December days are short and much of nature sleeps, it is still possible to experience its joys. Studies have shown that nature connection and wellbeing can still be boosted by continuing to notice the good things around us over the winter months, even in everyday places close to home. This research also found that time spent in nature doesn't need to increase – good news on short, cold days. Nature connection is built on engagement, actively noticing, in the park, at the bus stop or anywhere else you go during your daily routine. So, keep on noticing.

### *Activity*: A Christmas craft walk

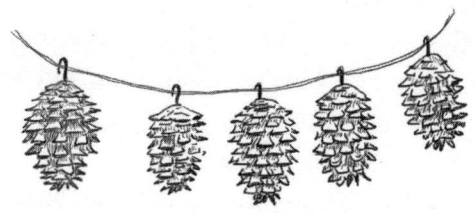

Christmas is a time for decorations and gifts. You can turn to nature for both. Think how you might bring a touch of nature to a day otherwise bent on consumption and reduce needless plastic, while being appreciated for your creativity!

Of course, it is also possible to turn to nature for other religious festivals. For example, you can celebrate Diwali, the Hindu Festival of Lights, with orange marigolds and lanterns made from gourds. And you can use colourful spring flowers to help celebrate Vaisakhi.

This activity involves a search for natural treasures

you can use to decorate your home and make gifts. A park or woodland is an ideal location for your craft walk; all you need is a bag, gloves and imagination. Remember to keep to paths and avoid uprooting plants or disturbing hibernating wildlife.

As you wander, look for fallen bits and pieces that you could add to your tree or use to bring a touch of nature into your home. Fill a glass vase with acorns, beechnuts or conkers, or scatter a few pine cones to make a simple decoration for a table or mantelpiece. Make rustic stars by tying twigs with ribbons, or if you're feeling more adventurous, have a go at creating a garland by shaping bendy hazel or willow switches to create a circle and then intertwining it with colourful leaves, dry seed pods, pine cones and rose hips, for a touch of red. Let nature inspire you, and don't be afraid to experiment.

Only use items that you are confident are safe. Some leaves, such as ivy, can irritate the skin and cause some people to have an allergic reaction, so be careful when handling them and where they are used, especially when young children are present.

Remember the head, heart and hand framework as you assemble your creations. Whatever the results, the sensory engagement is another step to connection. If your designs work well, they can become a meaningful part of your festivities.

## A nature connected society

Throughout the year, our nature connection journey has focused mainly on us as individuals, rather than on community-wide activity. However, the twin crises of biodiversity loss and warming climate require a new relationship with nature on a far larger scale. The root cause of both crises is a dominant, controlling relationship with nature, which is deeply embedded into our way of life. Our schooling, health services, transport systems and even housing form a web of disconnection it is difficult to escape.

Changing how we relate to the rest of the natural world is a challenge, and one in which we all have a role to play. We need people with a close connection with nature to lead the way in shaping the future of our institutions, structures and processes, so we can integrate nature connection into education, town planning and health and social care systems. Only this can bring the large-scale social and cultural shifts needed to meet the challenges we face.

Ultimately, we need our institutions to change their goals. For it is these goals that influence the design of our organisations and social structures and inform the standards and policies we live by each day. They also shape the information we're presented with. News and advertisements are feedback loops that sustain the current way of being. We all live and work within these systems and we need to do all we can to bring about a more nature-connected future.

Ultimately, there can be no human wellbeing without nature's wellbeing, so we have to be good ancestors. Often, a more sustainable future feels like it must be achieved by having things taken away. But, as we've seen, forging a relationship with nature is about anything but loss; rather, it leads to greater personal fulfilment and a thriving environment.

### *Activity*: A vision of the future

Transformational change requires the creation of new visions and opportunities for communities to take action. The first step is to imagine what a close relationship with nature within a modern technological society looks like. One where people are inspired to live from, in, with and *as* nature, in a community they want to be part of.

Imagine that you have been transported to the year 2040. Society has undergone a transformative shift and the evidence and practices in this book are mainstream in everyday life. Consider what your neighbourhood, community or town would be like. Consider all the elements: homes, businesses, shops, leisure, transport, schools and health.

Here are a few broad ideas to get your started:

- The value of our currency is pegged to the richness of our biodiversity.
- Our neighbourhoods, schools, parks and gardens

are rich landscapes, full of opportunities for meaningful engagement with nature on everyone's doorstep.

- Local arts organisations celebrate nature and a connection with it.
- A small levy on advertising is used to help people understand the value of nature for keeping well such that they turn to nature first for everyday wellbeing and leisure.
- Our relationship with nature is a running theme through education.
- People have a closer connection to what they eat, in terms of food miles, natural ingredients and growing.
- Nature itself has been given rights and a voice, with its interests and needs taken into consideration in decision-making processes.
- There is a harmonious coexistence between humans and the rest natural world.

*Activity*: **Get to know a tree**

Round off the year by observing your chosen tree in its winter form. See how it stands against the cold. Notice if it provides shelter for birds, how rain patterns its trunk, or if its branches are outlined by frost. Reflect on the full cycle of the seasons, the opening of its buds, the joy of its vibrant summer and its transition into autumn.

As you complete your nature journal, write a letter to

this tree as if it were a friend. Why do you like it? What has been the most memorable time this year? What do you want to say to this tree? Then write a reply from the tree. Think about the tree's likes, interests, wellbeing and life. Did the tree notice you? How did it feel? What wisdom does it have to share?

A project in Canada gave the opportunity for people to text a tree and receive a reply from a volunteer voicing the tree, and giving it its own personhood.[31] It was based on Mi'kmaw tradition, from the First Nations peoples of the Northeastern Woodlands of Canada. Over 10,000 messages were received. Respondents noted their trees' beauty and were grateful for their shade. The project was found to increase people's connection to trees.

## Angel: The waxwing

Through the months we have focused on all sorts of common birds – what I refer to as the angels from an extinction. The December angel is trickier to find. The waxwing is an exotic-looking bird, which tends to visit the UK in small numbers, but is a real gift when spotted. When it does arrive, it can be found in urban locations like supermarket car parks, where it is after the berries on rowan trees and hawthorns. Some years bring 'waxwing winters' when the birds arrive in greater numbers from Scandinavia and Russia if food there is scarce. Waxwings are about the size of a starling, reddish-brown in colour, with a crest, distinctive black face markings and red-tipped wings. All birds bring joy, but knowing something is a little more unusual makes it extra special.

## *For nature*: Plant a native tree – and celebrate!

December is a great time to plant a native tree. A gift for yourself, your family, community, future generations and the natural world. Plan a way to mark the occasion. Gather family and friends, to celebrate the moment. Sing songs and toast the tree's good health; perhaps ring a bell to mark the significance. A new tree in a community space or on the land of an obliging landowner would make a fine yearly tradition.

For now, we will assume you are planting your tree in a small space or garden. Here are a few possibilities:

- Wild cherry: a tree that can support both wildlife and nature connection activities with its fragrant spring blossom and edible cherries in summer.
- Rowan: an elegant tree that supports birds with its bright red berries.
- Holly: a classic for festive winter foliage, plus useful cover and berries for your local birds.
- Crab apple: another tree with beautiful spring blossom and small fruits in the autumn. It can

support a variety of wildlife.

- Hazel: this has attractive catkins and in autumn/winter provides nuts, so can attract wildlife.

Do some further research; a tree is a long-term commitment, so you need to be sure it is suitable for your site. Consider its fully grown size, the location of any power lines or buildings and any potential issues with the roots. You also need to choose a species that thrives in your local climate and conditions. If you don't have a garden, find out which trees can be planted in a large pot.

When you're ready to plant your tree:

1. Choose a spot. Find a location that receives at least a few hours of sunlight each day.
2. Dig a hole. It needs to be as deep as the root ball and twice as wide.
3. Plant your tree. Carefully remove the young sapling from its pot. Loosen any tightly bound roots and place it in the hole.
4. Fill the hole. Ensure the tree stands straight and fill the hole with the excavated soil. Tap the soil gently as you go to remove air pockets. Water well and often over the next spring and summer.
5. Celebrate!

# Closing a year of connection

Over a dozen years on, I can still vividly recall the closing of my first year of reconnection. Under a solid December sky, I revisited a narrow strip of replanted woodland, between a track and an airfield near where I live. As I walked, a sparrowhawk crossed my path low through the plantation. Rooks were about their nests and jackdaws jibed. There were very early signs of the new year to come, fresh hazel catkins hanging in still air. A magpie flew before me, its wings creating an orb of white around its darkness. As I continued along the long, straight, thin woodland, I was engulfed by a feeling beyond the limits of my language. I reached a patch of ancient wood pasture, where the oldest oak seemed to reflect my condition, like a mirror of my mind. I stopped and I stood in the landscape, until only the landscape remained.

During the year, we complete one orbit of the sun – our blue planet spinning all the while, one turn per day. Without knowing it, each of us trace a vast spiral through space and time. As my reconnection with nature grew, I imagined life and nature in patterns – at first, patterns of birdsong through the air, then the patterns mapped out by soaring swallows, until eventually I imagined matter coalescing around the patterns of rooks, flowers, trees and humans. The energy of life holding everything together and maintaining its form.

These grand thoughts remain deep in my mind, occasionally teased out by a passing rook or swift. What remains at the forefront of my nature connection is everyday joy. Every bird is a gift, every tree a fellow being, every flower a wilderness. These simple pleasures are embedded in my experience, and yet even now, modern life often wins the battle for my attention. Connecting with nature needs to be practised each day.

My hope is that you too have a story of reconnection to share; one that will sustain you for years to come. A story in which nature has become more than just an arena for recreation and is now an integral part of your being. A story you will share with your peers and across generations, and that you will apply both at leisure and in your work. The more people share their nature connection stories, the more easily we will live in harmony with nature. On a bountiful Earth, with plentiful song, and untroubled minds.

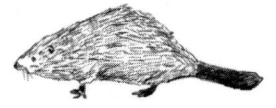

# Endnotes

1 Global Mind Project (2024) The Mental State of the World in 2023. https://mentalstateoftheworld.report/

2 Richardson, M., Hamlin, I., Elliott, L. R., & White, M. P. (2022). Country-level factors in a failing relationship with nature: Nature connectedness as a key metric for a sustainable future. *Ambio*, 51 (11), 2201–2213.

3 Martin, L., White, M. P., Hunt, A., et al. (2020). Nature contact, nature connectedness and associations with health, wellbeing and pro-environmental behaviours. *Journal of Environmental Psychology*, 68, 101389.

4 Lumber, R., Richardson, M., & Sheffield, D. (2017). Beyond knowing nature: contact, emotion, compassion, meaning, and beauty are pathways to nature connection. *PLoS One*, 12(5), e0177186. https://doi.org/10.1371/journal.pone.0177186

5 Barbett, L., Stupple, E., Sweet, M., & Richardson, M. (2019). An expert ranked list of pro-nature conservation behaviours for public use.

6 Kellert, S. R., & Wilson, E. O. (1993). *The Biophilia Hypothesis*. Island Press, Washington, DC.

7 Fanning, A. L., O'Neill, D. W., Hickel, J., & Roux, N. (2022). The social shortfall and ecological overshoot of nations. *Nature Sustainability*, 5(1), 26–36.

8 Li, H., Browning, M. H., Bardhan, M., Ying, M., Zhang, X., Cao, Y., & Zhang, G. (2024). Nature connectedness connects the visibility of trees through windows and mental wellbeing: a study on the "3 visible trees" component of the 3-30-300 rule. *International Journal of Environmental Health Research*, 1–13.

9 Vainio, K., Korrensalo, A., Takala, T., Räsänen, A., Lummaa, K., & Tuittila, E. S. (2024). Do you have a tree friend?—Human–tree relationships in Finland. *People and Nature*, 6(2), 646–659.

10 Richardson, M., & Hamlin, I. (2021). Nature engagement for human and nature's well-being during the Corona pandemic. *Journal of Public Mental Health*, 20(2), 83-93.

11 Ogletree, S. S., Huang, J. H., Reif, D., Yang, L., Dunstan, C., Osakwe, N., et al. & Hipp, J. A. (2023). The relationship between greenspace exposure and telomere length in the National Health and Nutrition Examination Survey. *Science of the Total Environment*, 905, 167452.

12 Kühn, S., Düzel, S., Eibich, P., et al. (2017). In search of features that constitute an 'enriched environment' in humans: associations between geographical properties and brain structure. *Scientific Reports*, 7, 11920.

13 Kesebir, S., & Kesebir, P. (2017). A growing disconnection from nature is evident in cultural products. *Perspectives on Psychological Science*, 12(2), 258–69.

14 Pirie, T. J., Thomas, R. L., & Fellowes, M. D. (2022). Pet cats (*Felis catus*) from urban boundaries use different habitats, have larger home ranges and kill more prey than cats from the suburbs. *Landscape and Urban Planning*, 220, 104338; Woods, M., McDonald, R. A., & Harris, S. (2003). Predation of wildlife by domestic cats *Felis catus* in Great Britain. *Mammal Review*, 33(2), 174–88; Marra, P. P. (2019). The ecological cost of pets. *Current Biology*, 29(19), R955–6; Trouwborst, A., McCormack, P. C., & Martínez Camacho, E. (2020). Domestic cats and their impacts on biodiversity: a blind spot in the application of nature conservation law. *People and Nature*, 2(1), 235–50.

15 Miller, S. G., Knight, R. L., & Miller, C. K. (2001). Wildlife responses to pedestrians and dogs. *Wildlife Society Bulletin*, 124–32; Banks, P. B., & Bryant, J. V. (2007). Four-legged friend or foe? Dog walking displaces native birds from natural areas.

*Biology Letters*, 3(6), 611–13.

16 Comber, C. A., & Dayer, A. A. (2022). Understanding attitudes and norms of dog walkers to reduce disturbances to shorebirds. *Human Dimensions of Wildlife*, 27(3), 236–250.

17 Dowling, B., & Weston, M. A. (1999). Managing a breeding population of the Hooded Plover *Thinornis rubricollis* in a high-use recreational environment. Bird Conservation International, 9(3), 255–270; Showler, D.A., Stewart, G.B., Sutherland,W.J. & Pullin, A.S. (2010). What is the impact of public access on the breeding success of ground-nesting and cliff-nesting birds? CEE review 05-010 (SR16).

18 Okin, G. S. (2017). Environmental impacts of food consumption by dogs and cats. *PloS one*, 12(8), e0181301; Pedrinelli, V., Teixeira, F. A., Queiroz, M. R., & Brunetto, M. A. (2022). Environmental impact of diets for dogs and cats. *Scientific Reports*, 12(1), 18510; European Environment Agency (2020). Average CO2 emissions from new cars and new vans increased again in 2019: https://www.eea.europa.eu/highlights/average-co2-emissions-from-new-cars-vans-2019

19 Gilbert, P. (ed.) (2005). *Compassion: Conceptualisations, Research and Use in Psychotherapy*. Hove: Routledge; Gilbert, P. (2014). The origins and nature of compassion focused therapy. *British Journal of Clinical Psychology*, 53, 6–41.

20 Lengieza, M. L. (2024). Eudaimonic self-expansion: The effects of eudaimonic reflections on nature connectedness. *Journal of Environmental Psychology*, 94, 102231.

21 Mochizuki-Kawai, H., Matsuda, I., & Mochizuki, S. (2020). Viewing a flower image provides automatic recovery effects after psychological stress. *Journal of Environmental Psychology*, 70, 101445.

22 Freud, S. (1949). *Civilization and its discontents*. London: Hogarth.

23 Passmore, H. A., & Holder, M. D. (2017). Noticing nature: Individual and social benefits of a two-week intervention. *The Journal of Positive Psychology*, 12(6), 537–546.

24 Barrable, A., & Booth, D. (2020). Green and Screen: Does Mobile Photography Enhance or Hinder Our Connection to Nature?. *Digital Culture & Education*, 12(2).

25 Piff, P. K., Dietze, P., Feinberg, M., Stancato, D. M., & Keltner, D. (2015). Awe, the small self, and prosocial behavior. *Journal of Personality and Social Psychology*, 108(6), 883.

26 Tagliazucchi, E., Roseman, L., Kaelen, M., Orban, C., Muthu-kumaraswamy, S. D., Murphy, K., et al. & Carhart-Harris, R. (2016). Increased global functional connectivity correlates with LSD-induced ego dissolution. *Current Biology*, 26(8), 1043-1050.

27 Tonello, L., Gashi, B., Scuotto, A., et al. (2018). The gastroin-testinal–brain axis in humans as an evolutionary advance of the root–leaf axis in plants: a hypothesis linking quantum effects of light on serotonin and auxin. *Journal of Integrative Neuroscience*, 17(2), 227–37.

28 Saarenpää, M., Roslund, M. I., Nurminen, N., Puhakka, R., Kummola, L., Laitinen, O. H., et al. & Sinkkonen, A. (2024). Urban indoor gardening enhances immune regulation and di-versifies skin microbiota—A placebo-controlled double-blinded intervention study. *Environment International*, 108705.

29 Renowden, C., Beer, T., & Mata, L. (2022). Exploring integrat-ed ArtScience experiences to foster nature connectedness through head, heart and hand. *People and Nature*, 4(2), 519–533.

30 Woolfson, E. (2010). *Corvus: A life with birds*. London: Granta Books.

31 Kass, J. S., Duinker, P. N., Zurba, M., & Smit, M. (2021). Test-ing a novel human-nature connection model with Halifax's urban forest using a text-messaging engagement strategy. *Urban Forestry & Urban Greening*, 65, 127350.

# Bibliography

Burton, C.M. and L.A. King. 2007. 'Effects of (very) brief writing on health: The two-minute miracle'. *British Journal of Health Psychology,* 13: 9–14. http://dx.doi.org/10.1348/135910707X250910

Chang, C. C., Lin, B. B., Feng, X., Andersson, E., Gardner, J., & Astell-Burt, T. (2024). A lower connection to nature is related to lower mental health benefits from nature contact. *Scientific Reports*, 14(1), 6705.

Menary, R. 2007. 'Writing as thinking'. *Language Sciences,* 29: 621–632. http://dx.doi.org/10.1016/j.langsci.2007.01.005

Passmore, H. A., & Holder, M. D. (2017). Noticing nature: Individual and social benefits of a two-week intervention. *The Journal of Positive Psychology*, 12(6), 537-546.

Pennebaker, J. W., & Seagal, J. D. (1999). Forming a story: The health benefits of narrative. *Journal of Clinical Psychology*, 55(10), 1243–1254.

Richardson, M., Hamlin, I., Elliott, L. R., & White, M. P. (2022). Country-level factors in a failing relationship with nature: Nature connectedness as a key metric for a sustainable future. *Ambio*, 51(11), 2201-2213.

Toepfer, S. M., & Walker, K. (2009). Letters of gratitude: Improving well-being through expressive writing. *Journal of Writing Research,* 1(3), 181–198.

## January

Camacho-Guzmán, A., Akerberg, V. D. Á., Martínez-Soto, J.,

Rodríguez-Soto, C., & Reyes, R. P. R. Connectedness to Nature, Well-Being and Presence of Birds.

Camacho-Guzmán, A., vila Akerberg, V. D. Ã., Martínez-Soto, J., Rodríguez-Soto, C., & Reyes, R. P. R. (2023). Connectedness to Nature, Well-Being and Presence of Birds. Fronteira: *Journal of Social, Technological and Environmental Science*, 12(1), 248–264

Li, H., Browning, M. H., Bardhan, M., Ying, M., Zhang, X., Cao, Y., & Zhang, G. (2024). Nature connectedness connects the visibility of trees through windows and mental wellbeing: a study on the "3 visible trees" component of the 3-30-300 rule. *International Journal of Environmental Health Research*, 1–13.

Liu, Y., Liu, J., Fan, X., Hu, Y., Guo, H., & Xue, F. (2024). Perceived birdsong diversity and restorativeness effect of soundscape: Interventions of birdsong audio and messaging. *Biodiversity Science*, 32(1), 23230.

Ratcliffe, E., Gatersleben, B., & Sowden, P. T. (2013). Bird sounds and their contributions to perceived attention restoration and stress recovery. *Journal of Environmental Psychology*, 36, 221–228.

Richardson, M. (2023). *Reconnection: Fixing our Broken Relationship with Nature*. Pelagic Publishing Ltd.

Richardson, M., & Hallam, J. (2013). Exploring the psychological rewards of a familiar semirural landscape: Connecting to local nature through a mindful approach. *The Humanistic Psychologist*, 41(1), 35–53.

Richardson, M., & Sheffield, D. (2017). Three good things in nature: Noticing nearby nature brings sustained increases in connection with nature. Psyecology, 8(1), 1–32.

Richardson, M., Hallam, J., & Lumber, R. (2015). One thousand good things in nature: Aspects of nearby nature associated with improved connection to nature. *Environmental Values*, 24(5), 603–619.

Seligman, M. E., Steen, T. A., Park, N., & Peterson, C. (2005). Positive psychology progress: empirical validation of interventions. *American Psychologist*, 60(5), 410.

White, M. E., Hamlin, I., Butler, C. W., & Richardson, M. (2023). The Joy of birds: The effect of rating for joy or counting garden bird species on wellbeing, anxiety, and nature connection. *Urban Ecosystems*, 1–11.

## February

Bang, M., Marin, A., Medin, D., & Washinawatok, K. (2015). Learning by observing, pitching in, and being in relations in the natural world. *In Advances in Child Development and Behavior*, 49, 303–13.

Cheung, S. S. (2015). Responses of the hands and feet to cold exposure. *Temperature*, 2(1), 105–120.

LeBlanc, J., Dulac, S., Cote, J., & Girard, B. (1975). Autonomic nervous system and adaptation to cold in man. *Journal of Applied Physiology*, 39(2), 181–186.

McEwan, K., Ferguson, F. J., Richardson, M., & Cameron, R. (2020). The good things in urban nature: A thematic framework for optimising urban planning for nature connectedness. *Landscape and Urban Planning*, 194, 103687.

McEwan, K., Richardson, M., Sheffield, D., Ferguson, F. J., & Brindley, P. (2019). A smartphone app for improving mental health through connecting with urban nature. *International Journal of Environmental Research and Public Health*, 16(18), 3373.

Richardson, M. (2023). Reconnection: Fixing our Broken Relationship with Nature. Pelagic Publishing Ltd.

Richardson, M., & Hamlin, I. (2021). Nature engagement for

human and nature's well-being during the Corona pandemic. *Journal of Public Mental Health*, 20(2), 83–93.

Richardson, M., Hamlin, I., Butler, C. W., Thomas, R., & Hunt, A. (2022). Actively noticing nature (not just time in nature) helps promote nature connectedness. *Ecopsychology*, 14(1), 8–16.

Richardson, M., Passmore, H. A., Lumber, R., Thomas, R., & Hunt, A. (2021). Moments, not minutes: The nature-wellbeing relationship. *International Journal of Wellbeing*, 11(1).

Russell, R., Guerry, A. D., Balvanera, P., Gould, R. K., Basurto, X., Chan, K. M., ... & Tam, J. (2013). Humans and nature: how knowing and experiencing nature affect well-being. *Annual Review of Environment and Resources*, 38, 473–502.

## March

Berto, R. (2014). The role of nature in coping with psycho-physiological stress: A literature review on restorativeness. *Behavioral Sciences*, 4(4), 39–409.

Birkett, L. P., & Newton-Fisher, N. E. (2011). How abnormal is the behaviour of captive, zoo-living chimpanzees? *PloS One*, 6(6), e20101.

Bowler, D. E., Buyung-Ali, L. M., Knight, T. M., & Pullin, A. S. (2010). A systematic review of evidence for the added benefits to health of exposure to natural environments. *BMC Public Health*, 10(1), 1–10.

Brüne, M., Brüne-Cohrs, U., McGrew, W. C., & Preuschoft, S. (2006) Psychopathology in great apes: concepts, treatment options and possible homologies to human psychiatric disorders. *Neuroscience & Biobehavioral Reviews*, 30(8), 1246–59.

Cameron, R. W. F., Brindley, P., Mears, M., et al. (2020). Where the wild things are! Do urban green spaces with greater avian biodiversity promote more positive emotions in humans? *Urban Ecosystems*. https://doi.org/10.1007/s11252-020-00929-z

Clarke, A. S., Juno, C. J., & Maple, T. L. (1982). Behavioral effects of a change in the physical environment: a pilot study of captive chimpanzees. *Zoo Biology*, 1(4), 371–80.

Ferdowsian, H. R., Durham, D. L., Kimwele, C., et al. (2011). Signs of mood and anxiety disorders in chimpanzees. *PloS One*, 6(6), e19855; Baker, C. (2021, December 13).

Hartig, T. et al. (2011). Health benefits of nature experience: psychological, social and cultural processes. In K. Nilsson, M. Sangster, C. Gallis, et al. (eds) Forests, Trees and Human Health (pp. 127–68). *Dordrecht: Springer*.

Joye, Y., & Bolderdijk, J. W. (2015). An exploratory study into the effects of extraordinary nature on emotions, mood, and prosociality. *Frontiers in Psychology*, 5, 1577.

Kellert, S. R., & Wilson, E. O. (1993). The Biophilia Hypothesis. Island Press, Washington, DC.

Kuo, M. (2015). How might contact with nature promote human health? Promising mechanisms and a possible central pathway. *Frontiers in Psychology*, 6, 1093

Lumber, R., Richardson, M., & Sheffield, D. (2017). Beyond knowing nature: contact, emotion, compassion, meaning, and beauty are pathways to nature connection. *PLoS One*, 12(5), e0177186. https://doi.org/10.1371/journal.pone.0177186

Martin, L., White, M. P., Hunt, A., et al. (2020). Nature contact, nature connectedness and associations with health, wellbeing and pro-environmental behaviours. *Journal of Environmental Psychology*, 68, 101389.

Methorst, J., Rehdanz, K., Mueller, T., et al. (2021). The importance of species diversity for human well-being in Europe. *Ecological Economics*, 181, 106917.

Pritchard, A., Richardson, M., Sheffield, D., & McEwan, K. (2020). The relationship between nature connectedness and eudaimonic well-being: A meta-analysis. *Journal of Happiness Studies*, 21, 1145–1167.

Richardson, M. (2023). Reconnection: Fixing our Broken Relationship with Nature. Pelagic Publishing Ltd.

Richardson, M., Maspero, M., Golightly, D., Sheffield, D., Staples, V., & Lumber, R. (2020). Nature: A new paradigm for well-being and ergonomics. *In New Paradigms in Ergonomics* (pp. 142–155). Routledge.

Sturm, V. E., Datta, S., Roy, A. R., Sible, I. J., Kosik, E. L., Veziris, C. R., ... & Keltner, D. (2022). Big smile, small self: Awe walks promote prosocial positive emotions in older adults. *Emotion*, 22(5), 1044. https://doi.org/10.1037/emo0000876

Swami, V., Barron, D., Weis, L., & Furnham, A. (2016). Bodies in nature: associations between exposure to nature, connectedness to nature, and body image in US adults. *Body Image*, 18, 153–61

Williams, K. J., Lee, K. E., Hartig, T., Sargent, L. D., Williams, N. S., & Johnson, K. A. (2018). Conceptualising creativity benefits of nature experience: Attention restoration and mind wandering as complementary processes. *Journal of Environmental Psychology*, 59, 36–45.

## April

Basu, A., Duvall, J., & Kaplan, R. (2019). Attention restoration theory: Exploring the role of soft fascination and mental bandwidth. *Environment and Behavior*, 51(9-10),

1055–1081.

BBC. (2021,). Households "buy 3.2 million pets in lock-down." BBC News. https://www.bbc.co.uk/news/business-56362987

Brantsæter, A. L., Ydersbond, T. A., Hoppin, J. A., Haugen, M., & Meltzer, H. M. (2017). Organic food in the diet: exposure and health implications. *Annual Review of Public Health*, 38, 295–313.

Cuff, M. (2022). What impact will planned new UK coal mine have on carbon emissions? New Scientist. https://www.newscientist.com/article/2350696-what-impact-will-planned-new-uk-coal-mine-have-on-carbon-emissions/

Egerer, M., Lin, B., Kingsley, J., Marsh, P., Diekmann, L., & Ossola, A. (2022). Gardening can relieve human stress and boost nature connection during the COVID-19 pandemic. *Urban Forestry & Urban Greening*, 68, 127483.

Franco, L. S., Shanahan, D. F., & Fuller, R. A. (2017). A review of the benefits of nature experiences: More than meets the eye. *International Journal of Environmental Research and Public Health*, 14(8), 864.

Fuhrman, J. (2018). The hidden dangers of fast and processed food. *American Journal of Lifestyle Medicine*, 12(5), 375–381.

Han, Y., & Xiao, H. (2020). Whole food–based approaches to modulating gut microbiota and associated diseases. *Annual Review of Food Science and Technology*, 11, 119–143.

Hewitt, A. (2017). The truth about cats' and dogs' environmental impact. UCLA. https://newsroom.ucla.edu/releases/the-truth-about-cats-and-dogs-environmental-impact

Lafferty, K. D., Goodman, D., & Sandoval, C. P. (2006). Restoration of breeding by snowy plovers following protection from disturbance. *Biodiversity & Conservation*, 15,

2217–2230.

Lee, K. E., Williams, K. J., Sargent, L. D., Williams, N. S., & Johnson, K. A. (2015). 40-second green roof views sustain attention: The role of micro-breaks in attention restoration. *Journal of Environmental Psychology*, 42, 182-189.

Niigaaniin, M., & MacNeill, T. (2022). Indigenous culture and nature relatedness: Results from a collaborative study. *Environmental Development*, 44, 100753.

Ohly, H., White, M. P., Wheeler, B. W., Bethel, A., Ukoumunne, O. C., Nikolaou, V., & Garside, R. (2016). Attention Restoration Theory: A systematic review of the attention restoration potential of exposure to natural environments. *Journal of Toxicology and Environmental Health*, Part B, 19(7), 305-343.

Pye, A., Bash, K., Joiner, A., & Beenstock, J. (2022). Good for the planet and good for our health: the evidence for whole-food plant-based diets. *BJPsych International*, 19(4), 90–92.

Richardson, M. (2023). *Reconnection: Fixing our Broken Relationship with Nature*. Pelagic Publishing Ltd.

Robin, L., Robin, K., Camerlenghi, E., Ireland, L., & Ryan-Colton, E. (2022). How Dreaming and Indigenous ancestral stories are central to nature conservation: Perspectives from Walalkara Indigenous Protected Area, Australia. *Ecological Management & Restoration*, 23, 43–52.

Robles, K. E., Gonzales-Hess, N., Taylor, R. P., & Sereno, M. E. (2023). Bringing nature indoors: characterizing the unique contribution of fractal structure and the effects of Euclidean context on perception of fractal patterns. *Frontiers in Psychology*, 14.

Srour, B., & Touvier, M. (2020). Processed and ultra-processed foods: coming to a health problem?. *International Journal* of *Food Sciences and Nutrition*, 71(6), 653–655.

Statista. (2024, February 13). Pet ownership in the UK 2009-2019. Statista. https://www.statista.com/statistics/308235/estimated-pet-ownership-in-the-united-kingdom-uk/

RHS. (n.d.). How gardeners can help our declining bees and other pollinators / RHS Gardening. Www.rhs.org.uk. https://www.rhs.org.uk/wildlife/help-our-declining-bees-and-other-pollinators

Uhlmann, K., Ross, H., Buckley, L., & Lin, B. B. (2022). Nature relatedness, connections to food and wellbeing in Australian adolescents. *Journal of Environmental Psychology*, 84, 101888.

Van den Berg, A. E., Joye, Y., & Koole, S. L. (2016). Why viewing nature is more fascinating and restorative than viewing buildings: A closer look at perceived complexity. *Urban Forestry & Urban Greening*, 20, 397–401.

Van Vliet, S., Beals, J. W., Martinez, I. G., Skinner, S. K., & Burd, N. A. (2018). Achieving optimal post-exercise muscle protein remodeling in physically active adults through whole food consumption. *Nutrients*, 10(2), 224.

Williams, K. J., Lee, K. E., Hartig, T., Sargent, L. D., Williams, N. S., & Johnson, K. A. (2018). Conceptualising creativity benefits of nature experience: Attention restoration and mind wandering as complementary processes. *Journal of Environmental Psychology*, 59, 36–45.

Langlois, M., & Chandon, P. (2024). Experiencing nature leads to healthier food choices. *Communications Psychology*, 2(1), 24.

**May**

Brown, K. W., & Ryan, R. M. (2003). The benefits of being present: mindfulness and its role in psychological well-being. *Journal of Personality and Social Psychology*, 84(4), 822.

Choe, E. Y., Jorgensen, A., & Sheffield, D. (2020). Does a natural environment enhance the effectiveness of Mindfulness-Based Stress Reduction (MBSR)? Examining the mental health and wellbeing, and nature connectedness benefits. *Landscape and Urban Planning*, 202, 103886.

Howell, A. J., Dopko, R. L., Passmore, H. A., & Buro, K. (2011). Nature connectedness: associations with well-being and mindfulness. *Personality and Individual Differences*, 51(2), 166–71.

Jones, R., Tarter, R., & Ross, A. M. (2021). Greenspace interventions, stress and cortisol: a scoping review. *International Journal of Environmental Research and Public Health*, 18(6), 2802.

Kobayashi, H., Song, C., Ikei, H., Park, B. J., Lee, J., Kagawa, T., & Miyazaki, Y. (2018). Forest walking affects autonomic nervous activity: a population-based study. *Frontiers in Public Health*, 6, 278.

Kotera, Y., Richardson, M., & Sheffield, D. (2020). Effects of shinrin-yoku (forest bathing) and nature therapy on mental health: A systematic review and meta-analysis. *International journal of mental health and addiction*, 1–25.

Lengieza, M. L. (2024). Eudaimonic self-expansion: The effects of eudaimonic reflections on nature connectedness. *Journal of Environmental Psychology*, 94, 102231.

Lengieza, M. L., & Swim, J. K. (2021). The paths to connectedness: A review of the antecedents of connectedness to nature. *Frontiers in Psychology*, 12, 763231.

Macaulay, R., Lee, K., Johnson, K., & Williams, K. (2022). Mindful engagement, psychological restoration, and connection with nature in constrained nature experiences.

*Landscape and Urban Planning*, 217, 104263.

Mao, G. X., Cao, Y. B., Yan, Y. A. N. G., Chen, Z. M., Dong, J. H., Chen, S. S., ... & Wang, G. F. (2018). Additive benefits of twice forest bathing trips in elderly patients with chronic heart failure. *Biomedical and Environmental Siences*, 31(2), 159–162.

McEwan, K. (2022). What is forest bathing? *Forest*, 2022, 06-28.

McEwan, K., Giles, D., Clarke, F. J., Kotera, Y., Evans, G., Terebenina, O., ... & Weil, D. (2021). A pragmatic controlled trial of forest bathing compared with compassionate mind training in the UK: Impacts on self-reported wellbeing and heart rate variability. *Sustainability*, 13(3), 1380.

McEwan, K., Potter, V., Kotera, Y., Jackson, J. E., & Greaves, S. (2022). 'This Is What the Colour Green Smells Like!': Urban Forest Bathing Improved Adolescent Nature Connection and Wellbeing. *International Journal of Environmental Research and Public Health*, 19(23), 15594.

Peterfalvi, A., Meggyes, M., Makszin, L., Farkas, N., Miko, E., Miseta, A., & Szereday, L. (2021). Forest bathing always makes sense: Blood pressure-lowering and immune system-balancing effects in late spring and winter in Central Europe. *International Journal of Environmental Research and Public Health*, 18(4), 2067.

Richardson, M. (2019). Beyond restoration: considering emotion regulation in natural well-being. *Ecopsychology*, 11(2), 123–129.

Richardson, M., & Sheffield, D. (2015). Reflective self-attention: A more stable predictor of connection to nature than mindful attention. *Ecopsychology*, 7(3), 166–175.

Richardson, M., McEwan, K., Maratos, F., & Sheffield, D. (2016). Joy and calm: How an evolutionary functional model of affect regulation informs positive emotions in nature. *Evolutionary Psychological Science*, 2, 308–320.

Subirana-Malaret, M., Miró, A., Camacho, A., Gesse, A., & McEwan, K. (2023). A Multi-Country Study Assessing the Mechanisms of Natural Elements and Sociodemographics behind the Impact of Forest Bathing on Well-Being. *Forests*, 14(5), 904.

Walker, H., Jena, A., McEwan, K., Evans, G., & Campbell, S. (2023). Natural Volatile Organic Compounds (NVOCs) Are Greater and More Diverse in UK Forests Compared with a Public Garden. *Forests*, 14(1), 92.

Hamann, G. A., & Ivtzan, I. (2017). 30 minutes in nature a day can increase mood, well-being, meaning in life and mindfulness: Effects of a pilot programme. *Social Inquiry into Well-being*, 2016, Vol. 2, No. 2.

**June**

Barton, J., Bragg, R., Pretty, J., Roberts, J., & Wood, C. (2016). The wilderness expedition: An effective life course intervention to improve young people's well-being and connectedness to nature. *Journal of Experiential Education*, 39(1), 59–72.

Greaney, S. (2022, June 15). Here comes the sun! Stonehenge and the summer solstice. The British Museum. https://www.britishmuseum.org/blog/here-comes-sun-stonehenge-and-summer-solstice

Greer, J. M. (2023, December 25). What Pagans can learn from Christianity. UnHerd. https://unherd.com/2023/12/what-pagans-can-learn-from-christianity/

Kamitsis, I., & Francis, A. J. (2013). Spirituality mediates the relationship between engagement with nature and psychological wellbeing. *Journal of Environmental Psychology*, 36,

136–143.

Kidner, D. W. (1994). Why psychology is mute about the environmental crisis. *Environmental Ethics*, 16(4), 359–76.

Lee, M. S., Park, B. J., Lee, J., Park, K. T., Ku, J. H., Lee, J. W., ... & Miyazaki, Y. (2013). Physiological relaxation induced by horticultural activity: transplanting work using flowering plants. *Journal of physiological anthropology*, 32(1), 1–5.

Passmore, H. A., & Krause, A. N. (2023). The Beyond-Human Natural World: Providing Meaning and Making Meaning. *International Journal of Environmental Research and Public Health*, 20(12), 6170.

Russell, R., Guerry, A. D., Balvanera, P., Gould, R. K., Basurto, X., Chan, K. M., ... & Tam, J. (2013). Humans and nature: how knowing and experiencing nature affect well-being. *Annual Review of Environment and Resources*, 38, 473–502.

Song, C., Igarashi, M., Ikei, H., & Miyazaki, Y. (2017). Physiological effects of viewing fresh red roses. *Complementary Therapies in Medicine, 35, 78–84*.

Trigwell, J. L., Francis, A. J., & Bagot, K. L. (2014). Nature connectedness and eudaimonic well-being: Spirituality as a potential mediator. *Ecopsychology, 6*(4), 241–251.

Williams, I. R., Rose, L. M., Raniti, M. B., et al. (2018). The impact of an outdoor adventure program on positive adolescent development: a controlled crossover trial. *Journal of Outdoor and Environmental Education*, 21(2), 207–36.

## July

Aminpour, P., Gray, S. A., Beck, M. W., et al. (2022). Urbanized knowledge syndrome – erosion of diversity and systems thinking in urbanites' mental models. *NPJ Urban*

*Sustainability*, 2(1), 1–10.

Arnberger, A., Schaper, S., Eder, R., & White, M. P. (2024). Visitor mood, restorativeness and connectedness to nature across four unmanaged urban outdoor swimming sites of varying naturalness. *Urban Forestry & Urban Greening*, 95, 128312.

Barrable, A., & Booth, D. (2020). Green and Screen: Does Mobile Photography Enhance or Hinder Our Connection to Nature?. *Digital Culture & Education*, 12(2).

Barrable, A., Wünsche, T. U., & Touloumakos, A. K. (2024). In "nature's embrace": Exploring connection to nature as experienced through wild swimming. Journal of Ecopsychology, 4, 2, 1-13. https://joe.nationalwellbeingservice.com/volumes/volume-4-2024/volume-4-article-2

Batool, A., Rutherford, P., McGraw, P., et al. (2021). Gaze correlates of view preference: comparing natural and urban scenes. Lighting Research & Technology, 14771535211055703;

Bingjing, C., Chen, G., & Shuhua, L. I. (2022). Looking at buildings or trees? Association of human nature relatedness with eye movements in outdoor space. *Journal of Environmental Psychology*, 101756.

Britton, E., Kindermann, G., Domegan, C., & Carlin, C. (2020). Blue care: A systematic review of blue space interventions for health and wellbeing. *Health Promotion International*, 35(1), 50–69.

Butler, C. W., Hamlin, I., Richardson, M., Lowe, M., & Fox, R. (2024). Connection for conservation: The impact of counting butterflies on nature connectedness and wellbeing in citizen scientists. *Biological Conservation*, 110497.

Denton, H., & Aranda, K. (2020). The wellbeing benefits of sea swimming. Is it time to revisit the sea cure? Qualitative

Research in Sport, *Exercise and Health*, 12(5), 647–663.

Douglas, J. W., & Evans, K. L. (2021). An experimental test of the impact of avian diversity on attentional benefits and enjoyment of people experiencing urban green-space. *People and Nature*. https://doi.org/10.1002/pan3.10279

Franĕk, M., Petružálek, J., & Šefara, D. (2019). Eye movements in viewing urban images and natural images in diverse vegetation periods. *Urban Forestry & Urban Greening*, 46, 126477.

Keltner, D., & Haidt, J. (2003). Approaching awe, a moral, spiritual, and aesthetic emotion. *Cognition and Emotion*, 17(2), 297–314.

Kesebir, S., & Kesebir, P. (2017). A growing disconnection from nature is evident in cultural products. *Perspectives on Psychological Science*, 12(2), 258–69.

McEwan, K., Richardson, M., Sheffield, D., Ferguson, F. J., & Brindley, P. (2019). A smartphone app for improving mental health through connecting with urban nature. *International Journal of Environmental Research and Public Health*, 16(18), 3373.

McEwan, K., Richardson, M., Sheffield, D., Ferguson, F. J., & Brindley, P. (2019). A smartphone app for improving mental health through connecting with urban nature. *International Journal of Environmental Research and Public Health*, 16(18), 3373.

Mears, M., Brindley, P., Barrows, P., Richardson, M., & Maheswaran, R. (2021). Mapping urban greenspace use from mobile phone GPS data. *Plos One*, 16(7), e0248622.

Pasanen, T. P., White, M. P., Wheeler, B. W., Garrett, J. K., & Elliott, L. R. (2019). Neighbourhood blue space, health and wellbeing: The mediating role of different types of physical activity. *Environment International*, 131, 105016.

Paxman, J. (2021). *Black Gold: The History of How Coal Made Britain*. London: William Collins.

Pocock, M. J., Hamlin, I., Christelow, J., Passmore, H. A., & Richardson, M. (2023). The benefits of citizen science and nature-noticing activities for well-being, nature connectedness and pro-nature conservation behaviours. *People and Nature*, 5(2), 591–606.

Richardson, M., Hamlin, I., Elliott, L. R., & White, M. P. (2022). Country-level factors in a failing relationship with nature: Nature connectedness as a key metric for a sustainable future. *Ambio*, 51(11), 2201–2213.

Richardson, M., Hussain, Z., & Griffiths, M. D. (2018). Problematic smartphone use, nature connectedness, and anxiety. *Journal of Behavioral Addictions*, 7(1), 109–116.

Rickard, S. C., & White, M. P. (2021). Barefoot walking, nature connectedness and psychological restoration: the importance of stimulating the sense of touch for feeling closer to the natural world. *Landscape Research*, 46(7), 975–991.

Sam, L. (2020). Nature as healer: A phenomenological study of the experiences of wild swimmers in Kenwood Ladies' Pond on Hampstead Heath. Consciousness, *Spirituality & Transpersonal Psychology*, 1, 34–48.

Schiebel, T., Gallinat, J., & Kühn, S. (2022). Testing the biophilia theory: automatic approach tendencies towards nature. *Journal of Environmental Psychology*, 79, 101725

Stehl, P., White, M. P., Vitale, V., Pahl, S., Elliott, L. R., Fian, L., & van den Bosch, M. (2023). From childhood blue space exposure to adult environmentalism: The role of nature connectedness and nature contact. *Journal of Environmental Psychology*, 102225.

Stellar, J. E., Gordon, A., Anderson, C. L., Piff, P. K., McNeil, G. D., & Keltner, D. (2018). Awe and humility. *Journal of*

*Personality and Social Psychology*, 114(2), 258.

Sturm, V. E., Datta, S., Roy, A. R., Sible, I. J., Kosik, E. L., Veziris, C. R., ... & Keltner, D. (2022). Big smile, small self: Awe walks promote prosocial positive emotions in older adults. *Emotion*, 22(5), 1044. https://doi.org/10.1037/emo0000876

Tagliazucchi, E., Roseman, L., Kaelen, M., Orban, C., Muthu-kumaraswamy, S. D., Murphy, K., ... & Carhart-Harris, R. (2016). Increased global functional connectivity correlates with LSD-induced ego dissolution. *Current Biology*, 26(8), 1043–1050.

Watts, L. (2019). An exploration of the pathways to nature connectedness evoked by wild swimming and walking in nature and the relationship of wild swimming and walking in nature to nature connectedness and subjective men-tal-wellbeing. Unpublished Masters Thesis.

White, M. P., Elliott, L. R., Gascon, M., Roberts, B., & Flem-ing, L. E. (2020). Blue space, health and well-being: A narrative overview and synthesis of potential benefits. *Environmental Research*, 191, 110169.

White, M. P., Elliott, L. R., Grellier, J., Economou, T., Bell, S., Bratman, G. N., ... & Fleming, L. E. (2021). Associations between green/blue spaces and mental health across 18 countries. *Scientific Reports*, 11(1), 8903.

**August**

Barnes, C., & Passmore, H. A. (2024). Development and test-ing of the Night Sky Connectedness Index (NSCI). *Journal of Environmental Psychology*, 93, 102198.

Berman, M. (1981). *The Reenchantment of the World*. Ithaca, NY: Cornell University Press.

Beute, F. & de Kort, Y. A. W. Salutogenic effects of the environment: review of health protective effects of nature and daylight. *Appl. Psychol. Health Well Being,* 6(1), 67–95 (2013).

Beute, F. & De Kort, Y. A. W. The natural context of wellbeing: Ecological momentary assessment of the influence of nature and daylight on affect and stress for individuals with depression levels varying from none to clinical. *Health Place,* 49, 7–18 (2018).

Beute, F., & de Kort, Y. A. (2013). Let the sun shine! Measuring explicit and implicit preference for environments differing in naturalness, weather type and brightness. *Journal of Environmental Psychology,* 36, 162–178.

Cartwright, B. D., White, M. P., & Clitherow, T. J. (2018). Nearby nature 'buffers' the effect of low social connectedness on adult subjective wellbeing over the last 7 days. *International Journal of Environmental Research and Public Health,* 15(6), 1238.

Chakraborty, U. (2020). Effects of different phases of the lunar month on living organisms. *Biological Rhythm Research,* 51(2), 254–282.

Diamond, J. (2013). *Guns, Germs and Steel: A Short History of Everybody for the Last 13,000 Years.* New York: Random House.

Drake, J. E. (2019). Examining the psychological and psychophysiological benefits of drawing over one month. *Psychology of Aesthetics, Creativity, and the Arts,* 13(3), 338.

Drake, J. E., Hastedt, I., & James, C. (2016). Drawing to distract: Examining the psychological benefits of drawing over time. *Psychology of Aesthetics, Creativity, and the Arts,* 10(3), 325.

Eisenstein, C. (2013). *The Ascent of Humanity: Civilization and the Human Sense of Self.* Berkeley, CA: North Atlantic

Books.

Foxon, A. (2022). *The Green Sketching Handbook: Relax, Unwind and Reconnect with Nature*. Pan Macmillan.

Hamilton, C. (2002). Dualism and sustainability. *Ecological Economics*, 42(1–2), 89–99.

Hill, S., Fischer, R., & Leong, L. Y. C. (2021). An empirical investigation of the relationship between nature engagement, connectedness with nature, and divergent-thinking creativity.

Leong, L. Y. C., Fischer, R., & McClure, J. (2014). Are nature lovers more innovative? The relationship between connectedness with nature and cognitive styles. *Journal of Environmental Psychology*, 40, 57–63.

Marlowe, F. W. (2005). Hunter-gatherers and human evolution. *Evolutionary Anthropology: Issues, News, and Reviews*, 14(2), 54–67;

Richardson, M. (2023). *Reconnection: Fixing our Broken Relationship with Nature*. Pelagic Publishing Ltd.

Russell, R., Guerry, A. D., Balvanera, P., Gould, R. K., Basurto, X., Chan, K. M., ... & Tam, J. (2013). Humans and nature: how knowing and experiencing nature affect well-being. *Annual Review of Environment and Resources*, 38, 473–502.

Schlebusch, C. M., Malmström, H., Günther, T., et al. (2017). Southern African ancient genomes estimate modern human divergence to 350,000 to 260,000 years ago. *Science*, 358(6363), 652–5.

Wyles, K. J., Pahl, S., Holland, M., & Thompson, R. C. (2017). Can beach cleans do more than clean-up litter? Comparing beach cleans to other coastal activities. *Environment and Behavior*, 49(5), 509–535.

**September**

Balding, M., & Williams, K. J. (2016). Plant blindness and the implications for plant conservation. *Conservation Biology*, 30(6), 1192–1199.

Bird-David, N. (1999). "Animism" revisited: personhood, environment, and relational epistemology. *Current Anthropology*, 40(S1), S67–S91.

Eisenstein, C. (2013). *The ascent of humanity: Civilization and the human sense of self.* North Atlantic Books.

Falk, J. H., & Balling, J. D. (2010). Evolutionary influence on human landscape preference. *Environment and Behavior*, 42(4), 479–493.

Hepburn, L., Smith, A. C., Zelenski, J., & Fahrig, L. (2021). Bird diversity unconsciously increases people's satisfaction with where they live. *Land*, 10(2), 153.

Kamitsis, I., & Francis, A. J. (2013). Spirituality mediates the relationship between engagement with nature and psychological wellbeing. *Journal of Environmental Psychology*, 36, 136–143.

Krosnick, S. E., Baker, J. C., & Moore, K. R. (2018). The pet plant project: Treating plant blindness by making plants personal. *The American Biology Teacher*, 80(5), 339–345.

Lengen, C. (2015). The effects of colours, shapes and boundaries of landscapes on perception, emotion and mentalising processes promoting health and well-being. *Health & Place*, 35, 166–177.

Naveh, D., & Bird-David, N. (2014). How persons become things: economic and epistemological changes among Nayaka hunter-gatherers. *Journal of the Royal Anthropological Institute*, 20(1), 74–92.

O'Driscall, D (2022). Introduction to Animism: Definitions and Core Practices for Nature Spirituality https://thedruidsgarden.com/2022/07/14/introduction-to-animism-definitions-and-core-practices-for-nature-spirituality/

Ojalehto Mays, B., Seligman, R., & Medin, D. L. (2020). Cognition beyond the human: Cognitive psychology and the new animism. *Ethos*, 48(1), 50–73.

Parsley, K. M. (2020). Plant awareness disparity: A case for renaming plant blindness. *Plants, People, Planet*, 2(6), 598–601.

Pritchard, A. (2024). The relationship between nature connectedness and eudaimonic wellbeing: the role of childhood nature experiences, perceptions of naturalness and biodiversity, and fascination and awe. Unpublished PhD Thesis.

Richardson, M., Hamlin, I., Elliott, L. R., & White, M. P. (2022). Country-level factors in a failing relationship with nature: Nature connectedness as a key metric for a sustainable future. *Ambio*, 51(11), 2201–2213.

Rottman, J., Crimston, C. R., & Syropoulos, S. (2021). Treehuggers versus human-lovers: Anthropomorphism and dehumanization predict valuing nature over outgroups. Cognitive Science, 45(4), e12967.

Shores, J., Daniel, B., & Faircloth, W. B. (2023). The Experience of Inspiration in Natural Landscapes: Awe, Wonder, Sublimity, and Bergson's Qualitative Multiplicity. *Journal of Experiential Education*, 10538259231205291.

Stevens, P. (2010). Embedment in the environment: A new paradigm for well-being?. P*erspectives in Public Health*, 130(6), 265–269.

Tam, K. P., Lee, S. L., & Chao, M. M. (2013). Saving Mr. Nature: Anthropomorphism enhances connectedness to and protectiveness toward nature. *Journal of Experimental Social Psychology*, 49(3), 514–521.

Tang, I. C., Sullivan, W. C., & Chang, C. Y. (2015). Perceptual evaluation of natural landscapes: The role of the individual connection to nature. *Environment and Behavior*, 47(6), 595–617.

Wyles, K. J., White, M. P., Hattam, C., Pahl, S., King, H., & Austen, M. (2019). Are some natural environments more psychologically beneficial than others? The importance of type and quality on connectedness to nature and psychological restoration. *Environment and Behavior*, 51(2), 111–143.

Zhang, M., Delgado-Baquerizo, M., Li, G., Isbell, F., Wang, Y., Hautier, Y., ... & Wang, L. (2023). Experimental impacts of grazing on grassland biodiversity and function are explained by aridity. *Nature communications*, 14(1), 5040.

## October

Bruni, C. M., Winter, P. L., Schultz, P. W., Omoto, A. M., & Tabanico, J. J. (2017). Getting to know nature: evaluating the effects of the Get to Know Program on children's connectedness with nature. *Environmental Education Research*, 23(1), 43–62.

Franco, L. S., Shanahan, D. F., & Fuller, R. A. (2017). A review of the benefits of nature experiences: More than meets the eye. *International Journal of Environmental Research and Public Health*, 14(8), 864.

Moula, Z., Palmer, K., & Walshe, N. (2022). A systematic review of arts-based interventions delivered to children and young people in nature or outdoor spaces: impact on nature connectedness, Health and Wellbeing. *Frontiers in Psychology*, 13, 858781.

Robinson, J. M. (n.d.). Why spending more time in nature

could reduce "germaphobia." The Conversation. https://theconversation.com/why-spending-more-time-in-nature-could-reduce-germaphobia-163741

Robinson, J. M., Breed, M., & Cameron, R. (n.d.). How the trees in your local park help protect you from disease. *The Conversation*. https://theconversation.com/how-the-trees-in-your-local-park-help-protect-you-from-disease-160312

Robinson, J. M., Cando-Dumancela, C., Antwis, R. E., et al. (2021). Exposure to airborne bacteria depends upon vertical stratification and vegetation complexity. *Scientific Reports*, 11(1), 1–16.

Sender, R., Fuchs, S., & Milo, R. (2016). Revised estimates for the number of human and bacteria cells in the body. PLoS Biology, 14(8), e1002533.

Van Gordon, W., Shonin, E., & Richardson, M. (2018). Mindfulness and nature. *Mindfulness*, 9(5), 1655–1658.

## November

Brambilla, E., Petersen, E., Stendal, K., Sundling, V., MacIntyre, T. E., & Calogiuri, G. (2024). Effects of immersive virtual nature on nature connectedness: A systematic review and meta-analysis. *Digital Health*, 10, 20552076241234639.

Cameron, R. W., Brindley, P., Mears, M., McEwan, K., Ferguson, F., Sheffield, D., ... & Richardson, M. (2020). Where the wild things are! Do urban green spaces with greater avian biodiversity promote more positive emotions in humans?. *Urban Ecosystems*, 23, 301–317.

Correia, R. A. (2024). Acknowledging and understanding the contributions of nature to human sense of time. *People and Nature*, 00, 1–9. https://doi.org/10.1002/pan3.10601

Deep Time Diligence – with Tyson Yunkaporta https://emergencemagazine.org/interview/deep-time-diligence/

Harper, L & Fawcett, K. (2024). Can botanical folk tales help to reduce plant awareness disparity and aid plant conservation efforts? Unpublished manuscript.

Hughes, K., & Moscardo, G. (2024). Once upon a time: the impact of storytelling on connecting people to natural landscapes. *Environmental Education Research*, 30(2), 235–250.

Kahn Jr, P. H., Friedman, B., Gill, B., Hagman, J., Severson, R. L., Freier, N. G., ... & Stolyar, A. (2008). A plasma display window?—The shifting baseline problem in a technologically mediated natural world. *Journal of Environmental Psychology*, 28(2), 192–199.

Lengieza, M. L., & Richardson M. (2024). *Situation Networks: The emotions, activities, and features that are central to nature-connectedness experiences.*

Leung, G. Y., Hazan, H., & Chan, C. S. (2022). Exposure to nature in immersive virtual reality increases connectedness to nature among people with low nature affinity. *Journal of Environmental Psychology*, 83, 101863.

Pasca, L., Carrus, G., Loureiro, A., Navarro, Ó., Panno, A., Tapia Follen, C., & Aragonés, J. I. (2022). Connectedness and well-being in simulated nature. Applied Psychology: *Health and Well-Being*, 14(2), 397–412.

Ray, N. M., & McCain, G. (2012). Personal identity and nostalgia for the distant land of past: Legacy tourism. International *Business & Economics Research Journal* (IBER), 11(9), 977–990.

Routledge C., Arndt, J., Wildschut, T., Sedikides, C., Hart, C., Juhl, J., Vingerhoets, A. J., & Scholtz, W. (2011). The past makes the present meaningful: Nostalgia as an existential resource. *Journal of Personality and Social Psychology*, 101,

638–652.

Spangenberger, P., Freytag, S. C., & Geiger, S. M. (2024). Embodying nature in immersive virtual reality: Are multisensory stimuli vital to affect nature connectedness and pro-environmental behaviour?. *Computers & Education*, 212, 104964.

Van Tilburg, W. A., Sedikides, C., Wildschut, T., & Vingerhoets, A. J. (2019). How nostalgia infuses life with meaning: From social connectedness to self-continuity. *European Journal of Social Psychology*, 49(3), 521–532.

Yeo, N. L., White, M. P., Alcock, I., Garside, R., Dean, S. G., Smalley, A. J., & Gatersleben, B. (2020). What is the best way of delivering virtual nature for improving mood? An experimental comparison of high definition TV, 360 video, and computer generated virtual reality. *Journal of Environmental Psychology*, 72, 101500.

Van Gordon, W., Shonin, E., & Richardson, M. (2018). Mindfulness and nature. *Mindfulness*, 9(5), 1655–1658.

**December**

Coughlan, A., Ross, E., Nikles, D., De Cesare, E., Tran, C., & Pensini, P. (2022). Nature guided imagery: An intervention to increase connectedness to nature. *Journal of Environmental Psychology*, 80, 101759.

Richardson, M., Dobson, J., Abson, D. J., Lumber, R., Hunt, A., Young, R., & Moorhouse, B. (2020). Applying the pathways to nature connectedness at a societal scale: a leverage points perspective. *Ecosystems and People*, 16(1), 387 401.

McEwan, K., Richardson, M., Sheffield, D., Ferguson, F. J., & Brindley, P. (2019). A smartphone app for improving mental health through connecting with urban nature. International journal of environmental research and public health, 16(18), 3373.

Muneghina, O., Van Gordon, W., Barrows, P., & Richardson, M. (2021). A novel mindful nature connectedness intervention improves paranoia but not anxiety in a nonclinical population. *Ecopsychology*, 13(4), 248–256.

Passmore, H. A., Yargeau, A., & Blench, J. (2022). Wellbeing in winter: Testing the Noticing Nature Intervention during winter months. *Frontiers in Psychology*, 13, 840273.

Schaal, T., Mitchell, M., Scheele, B. C., Ryan, P., & Hanspach, J. (2023). Using the three horizons approach to explore pathways towards positive futures for agricultural landscapes with rich biodiversity. *Sustainability Science*, 18(3), 1271–1289.

Sharpe, B., Hodgson, A., Leicester, G., Lyon, A., & Fazey, I. (2016). Three horizons: a pathways practice for transformation. *Ecology and Society*, 21(2).

# Appendix and Further Reading

*An expert ranked list of pro-nature conservation behaviours.*

We asked 70 conservation experts to review a long list of conservation behaviours for their ecological impact – ones that are worth encouraging. The menu below includes all the things you can do that most experts agreed on. The star rating shows those which were seen as the most beneficial for nature. These are things you can do at home, in your garden or other land you have access to.

| | |
|---|---|
| Put up nest boxes for birds | *** |
| Put up a bat box | *** |
| Provide food for birds and wildlife | *** |
| When out in nature, try to avoid disturbing wildlife | *** |
| Provide water for birds and wildlife | *** |
| Plant pollinator-friendly plants | *** |
| Leave an undisturbed area for wildlife | *** |
| Install hedgehog holes to help wildlife move about | *** |
| Have a wildflower area | *** |
| Avoid using insecticides | *** |
| Have a wildlife pond | *** |
| Leave log piles as homes for wildlife | *** |
| Put up a bee hotel | *** |
| Grow plants with berries/fruits | *** |
| Get a hedgehog home | *** |
| Plant native plants | *** |

| Grow plants with different flowering seasons | *** |
| Pick up litter | ** |
| Plant a tree | ** |
| Avoid removing native hedges | ** |
| Avoid using weed killer | ** |
| Avoid installing artificial turf | * |
| Avoid using synthetic fertiliser | * |
| Avoid removing green space for hard standing | * |
| Compost at home | * |

## Further reading

Should you wish to delve much deeper into the science of nature connection you may be interested in the author's book *Reconnection: Fixing our broken relationship with nature.*

# Acknowledgments

This book was written across evenings and weekends, squirrelled away in a writing shed overlooking a field, in six enjoyable months. During that time, many birds perched in the hawthorn a few feet away from the window, bringing joy, calm and company. Writing this book has emphasised the power of nature further than I imagined. I finished writing it on a sunny day in the glorious month of May. Each spring is more precious than the last. I extend my deepest gratitude to the web of life in the more than human world and to you the reader for your desire to connect more deeply with that world. I'd also like to thank the staff at New River Books for the idea and opportunity, and to Aurea in particular for the helpful comments and swift progress. Special thanks also to my family, Liz, Leon and Isla, who reviewed all or parts of the first draft. And to Mike Lengieza for a full review and providing inspiration over a pint of Jaipur at the fabulous Exeter Arms.

# NATURE NOTES

# NATURE NOTES

# NATURE NOTES

# NATURE NOTES

## NATURE NOTES

# NATURE NOTES

# NATURE NOTES